DETOUR

A Roadmap For When Life Gets Rerouted

May you see opportunity in your adversity!

Cam

Cam Taylor

Detour
Copyright © 2017 by Cam Taylor

Cover design by Bitty Berlinghoff
Layout by Cam Taylor
Editing by James R. Coggins

Scripture quotations marked NLT are taken from the Holy Bible, New Living Translation, copyright © 1996, 2004, 2007 by Tyndale House Foundation. Used by permission of Tyndale House Publishers, Inc., Carol Stream, Illinois 60188. All rights reserved. Scripture quotations marked NIV are taken from the Holy Bible, New International Version®, NIV® Copyright ©1973, 1978, 1984, 2011 by Biblica, Inc.® Used by permission. All rights reserved worldwide. Scripture quotations marked MSG are taken from The Message (MSG). Copyright © 1993, 1994, 1995, 1996, 2000, 2001, 2002 by Eugene H. Peterson.

Published in Canada by Infocus Publishing (camtaylor.net/publishing)
3731 Millar Court
Abbotsford, BC V2S 7K5

ISBN 978-0-9950968-6-8

This book is dedicated to my family, friends, and the host of people who helped make this journey possible.

And to Vicky,
my constant companion and friend from start to finish.

Table of Contents

Introduction: The Day the Lights Went Out

I had no idea what had happened to me, but one thing I knew for sure—no matter how hard I tried to wake up, I couldn't do it. But the questions remained: "How did I end up in this land of fog where everyone seems to be dressed in white? Who turned out the lights? Why am I stuck in this dream?"

It wasn't until two days later that I started to piece together the story of what had happened that day.

"What a great day for a ride," I told myself that sunny Saturday morning. My wife Vicky and I had been anticipating this day for several weeks, knowing that in British Columbia's Lower Fraser Valley the middle of April is a great time to license the bike and get back on the road for some riding pleasure.

One of the reasons I enjoyed summer so much was the memories we created on our road trips. Putting on the leathers, shining up the bike, planning the route, and riding in the open air— it was all high on our summer to do list. We had folders full of pictures and hearts full of memories from this hobby we loved.

The plan for our first ride of the season was a simple one—ride from our house to Harrison Hot Springs (about forty minutes away). Once at Harrison, we would view the lake, drink a hot cup of Americano, breathe in a few whiffs of fresh mountain air, and then head back home in time for supper. At least, that was our plan.

What started out as a picture perfect day would not end that way. At roughly 1:45 p.m., I closed the garage door, mounted the bike with Vicky, and rode off into the sunshine. At approximately 2:30 p.m., the lights went out.

As we cruised along Highway 7 close to the small town of Deroche, a Cavalier approached the highway from our right. The driver intended to make an uneventful left-hand turn onto the highway and go off to enjoy his afternoon cup of soup at a local restaurant before starting his shift at a local dairy farm. Instead of taking the necessary precautions, the driver of the Cavalier looked to the right but failed to look left. He pulled out right in front of us. Having no place to go, I slammed on the brakes, laid twenty feet of rubber, and then laid the bike down. In the blink of an eye, the bike had bounced off the side of the car. My broken body was left pinned under the engine, and Vicky was lying in pain on the shoulder of the road.

As you can imagine, this accident scene created quite a stir on that country road. In seconds, people started arriving from all directions. I was groaning in pain and asking for someone to lift the car off my head while Vicky was coming to realize her leg was bent awkwardly in front of her face.

Second on the scene was an acquaintance from our church, Tom Cassel. He didn't realize it was me under the car because he couldn't see my face behind the helmet. But, being the caring person he was, he proceeded to comfort and support me while I lay there broken and in a state of shock. Tom had the shock of his life when, the next day in church, he saw our faces flash onto the screen with a request to pray for us.

While lying there on the pavement, all I can remember is feeling as if a heavy, warm fog had settled in all around me. The lights were out, and I felt no pain.

Eventually, a helicopter came, and the paramedics stabilized our broken bodies as best they could. They assessed the damage and determined the best way to move us safely was by helicopter, with the destination being Royal Columbian Hospital (RCH) in New Westminster, B.C. RCH was chosen because it was the trauma hospital for our region.

It had become clear that my injuries were life-threatening, as a large quantity of blood had already been lost due to internal hemorrhaging. The compound fracture of my right femur was also a big concern. After our leathers and clothing were cut off, we were strapped to backboards, loaded into the helicopter, and flown away to RCH. The last time I had taken a helicopter ride was to see the scenery. This time, all I saw was darkness. I kept wishing that someone would turn the lights back on.

There were many prayers offered that night, and there was much anxiety in the hearts and minds of our family and friends. The hospital staff did what they do best. They attended to our wounds, ran a battery of tests, and got us stabilized for the night. The next day, we underwent the surgeries necessary to put our broken bones back together with the necessary pins, plates, and screws so we could start the long road of healing and recovery.

So, who turned out the lights? I began to learn the answer to that question two days later when I woke up out of the darkness. The first thing I remember is my two kids, Caleb and Elena, standing over my bed in the intensive care unit (ICU) with tentative smiles on their faces. As the lights slowly came on, I heard the story of how our ride had ended abruptly that Saturday afternoon.

It took a few days for the full impact of that traumatic event to sink in. I did not know at the time how long and arduous the journey would be. One thing was true, however—at least, I would take it with the lights on.

Why I Wrote This Book

I wrote this book to help people prepare for and navigate adversity and the setbacks that come in life. The content for this book came largely from the blogging I did during my recovery. The theme for that blog was: "Hoping for the best and dancing with the rest."

The process of writing turned into daily therapy. It gave my life purpose and resulted in considerable personal growth. The writing also gave me something to do while I waited for my detour to end. Initially I wrote to help myself, but eventually I realized that what I was learning might also help others who were on their own detours.

A new word I discovered was "opporversity." It may not be in the dictionary, but it has a definite meaning: "the thriving partnership between opportunity and adversity." That word said to me, "Instead of trying to get out of your adverse situation prematurely, decide to lean into the challenge and search for a deeper purpose while on the road you've been asked to travel." I said, "OK."

This book looks at adversity, perseverance, change, recovery, forgiveness, suffering, grief, and a host of other themes that describe our experience when life is rerouted. Everything I talk about in this book was lived out in my personal experience.

Whether you are on a detour now, have been on one, know someone who is on one, or need to prepare for an upcoming detour (which is going to come, sooner or later, by the way), this book is for you. My hope is that you will be encouraged by my story, find a connection to your own story, and be able to take the steps necessary to keep growing and moving forward.

Part 1: The Road Ends

This book has three parts. The first part is about the call to go on a journey we were not expecting yet have been asked to travel. I use the metaphor of a detour because it represents what adversity, loss, and hardship can feel like. Our life is going along just fine, and then, all of a sudden, the road ends. A sign reads, "You can't go this way but must take a detour."

When our accident happened, I was asked to step off the road I was on and divert my course immediately. The road had ended without warning, and I was forced to redirect my course.

When the road ended, I was forced to give up control, find hope when hope seemed lost, and live with a new level of uncertainty. The plans I had were shelved, and I had to make daily choices to keep walking with faith into an unknown future.

Chapter 1: Control

You may think it's true, but it isn't. The last two lines of the poem "Invictus" by William Ernest Henley say: "I am the master of my fate; I am the captain of my soul." These words couldn't be further from the truth.

Now, on one level, we do have control. We make choices that have predetermined consequences. We guide our own vessel through stormy and calm seas to a predetermined destination. We take initiative. We lead people. We go about living. But (and it's a very big but) if you think you "actually" control the outcome of where your life will go or not go on any given day, that's a problem.

My "I'm not in control" story

It was a beautiful Saturday morning. The weather forecast was for sun and warmer weather, the first we'd had after a long, damp winter. Our plan was coming together. It started with a morning run and then a trip to Superstore with Vicky for our weekly grocery shop. After we returned home, I went down to the insurance office to buy six months of insurance for our 750 Honda Shadow motorcycle. Plenty of summer riding pleasure lay ahead.

Now, I didn't think about it at the time, but in my subconscious I was assuming things that day would go according to my plan. After all, I had been riding for twenty years without incident. Vicky and I wore the proper riding gear, I had learned defensive driving skills, and I watched every car in sight for the slightest hint that we had not been seen. I had learned to control my reactions and actions while driving my motorcycle, so I was in control, right?

Unfortunately, at 2:30 p.m. on April 23, 2011, the control myth I adhered to was shattered—and so was I. I probably did see the Cavalier that turned into our path from a side road, but the driver did not see me, and there was nothing I could do to stop what was about to happen.

The counterpoint

You and I do not control our lives. We do not control with certainty the outcome of any given day. We make plans. We try our best to stay out of trouble, eat healthy, make wise decisions, and drive safely, but unfortunately (or fortunately) we are not actually in control.

Who is really in control? Is God? If he is, what's your reaction to that news? Do you get angry and quit reading? Do you look up at God and say, "If you are in control, why don't you stop the suffering, the accidents, and all the pain in the world?" That's a reasonable question in light of our tendency to blame someone else for our lack of control.

As I reflected on our out-of-control reality, I came to the following realization: We live in a broken world where stuff happens that is outside our control. Therefore, our best option is to put our trust in a reliable God who lives outside of time and keeps our best interest in mind in the long run—the eternal long run.

This perspective does not answer every question or satisfy every "why" you and I struggle with, but it does take the pressure off our need to always be in control. Another perspective that helps us to overcome our desire to be in control is to learn to tell time other than by a clock.

Learning to tell time

The ancient Greeks had two words for time—*chronos* and *kairos*. Our ability to be more comfortable with a lack of control is influenced by our ability to set our clock to the time that best serves a life out of control.

Chronos time is defined as something we measure with a stopwatch. It's what we race against and number our days by.

Kairos, on the other hand, defines time as something we measure with a heart rate monitor. *Kairos* time is movement that can't be counted. It is more about seasons and less about days.

Both *chronos* and *kairos* have a place. However, when we are rocked by adversity, loss, and life-altering circumstances, what is important is the ability to tell *kairos* time.

Solomon used the language of *kairos* when he wrote: "There is a time for everything, and a season for every activity under the heavens: a time to be born and a time to die, a time to plant and a time to uproot, a time to kill and a time to heal, a time to tear down and a time to build, a time to weep and a time to laugh, a time to mourn and a time to dance…"[1]

An out-of-control life appeared where the road ended

When the crash occurred, time stood still. For two days, I was heavily medicated so I wouldn't wake up. When I did wake up, I realized very quickly that the life I thought I had by the tail was now beyond my control. Not only had I been unable to stop the accident, I couldn't stop all the consequences that would come next.

My life before the accident was measured. I had plans—seminars to lead, people to help, bike trips to take. After the accident, all my plans were put on hold. I was on God's timetable, thrown into unmeasured *kairos* time. My neatly packaged, well-planned life had been tossed up into the air, blown apart, and scattered randomly across the landscape.

Kairos moments are opportunities that take us places in our minds and hearts that we cannot reach when we live on *chronos* time. After the accident, my life was no longer governed by the clock and the need to get things done on time. Things had changed drastically, and where the big and little hands were sitting did not matter.

We will never plumb the full depth of human experience if we live only on controlled *chronos* time. It is *kairos* time that opens up the door to new discoveries about ourselves, our world, our God, and what really matters in life. Embracing *kairos* time changes everything.

Know when your out-of-control life needs some *kairos* time

You need *kairos* time when you're feeling bewildered and lost. You need *kairos* time when you wake up somewhere between an ending and a new beginning. You need *kairos* time when your dreams have been crushed or put on hold. You need *kairos* time when a loss has left you reeling with pain and numbness.

Many of life's experiences don't fit neatly into a calendar. They play out on their own terms, and, in the process, they teach us multiple life lessons. In the midst of these experiences, if you fight living on *kairos* time, you will only increase your stress and frustration level. On the other hand, if you accept the opportunity to live on *kairos* time, it will open windows through which new insights and transforming thoughts can stream into your life. You will gain a "*kairos* perspective."

Four ways I learned to live on *kairos* time

1. I prayed almost every day the following words: "God, grant me the serenity to accept the things I cannot change, the courage to change the things I can, and the wisdom to know the difference." This is called the Serenity Prayer, and it was my friend when life was out of control.

2. I connected with my greater purpose and used it as a filter to find traction when events and circumstances were beyond my control. I'm not sure where I would have been without a purpose to look up to.

3. I learned to have the mind and teachability of a child. A child learns to walk by tripping over obstacles, falling down, getting back up, making some adjustments, then starting to walk again.

4. I exercised my faith muscle and learned on a whole new level to trust a personal God who had my best interest at heart. I realized how little I really knew, and I embraced the opportunity to learn those deeper life lessons that could only be learned when life was out of control and made no sense.

Detour Reflections

❖ Think about times when you thought you were in control but discovered you really weren't.

❖ What part of your life needs to be governed more by *kairos* time than by *chronos* time?

Chapter 2: Hope

It has been said that "Man can live forty days without food, three days without water, eight minutes without air, but only one second without hope." True hope is essential for life. False hope, or wishful thinking, is not enough. False hope says, "I hope it rains tomorrow"—without any clouds on the horizon to back up that claim. True hope contains an expectation for something to occur in the future, along with grounds for believing it will in fact happen.

How I found true hope when the road ended

The days leading up to my accident were filled with hope and promise. I had purpose and direction and was engaged in meaningful activity. I was excited about what lay ahead and had a plan to get there. When I woke up on April 25, 2011, I found myself lying helplessly in the ICU, with my hopes dashed.

Lying there, I was confused, in excruciating pain, and scrambling to find my bearings. Between naps, painkillers, blood tests, and nurses turning me over to prevent bed sores, I asked questions. I wondered, "When will I get back to doing what I love to do? When will I run, coach, travel, walk? When will I be normal again?"

Initially, my expectation was for a speedy recovery. I expected to be walking in eight weeks. I expected to be back to work in three or four months. I expected to be running by September. I expected to be working internationally before the end of the year.

The grounds for those expectations were the words expressed by doctors, physiotherapists, and other experts who presumably knew what they were talking about (as well as some of my own wishful thinking). Sure, they left the door open for some possible worst case scenarios, but I didn't for a second think those scenarios would happen.

My hope included both future expectations and grounds for believing those expectations would come to pass. But I was wrong, very wrong.

When hope loses its ground

My recovery went well for a while, but everything changed just a few short months later. The hope I had lost traction. The signs had been there earlier on in my recovery, but since I was naive and had no experience with infection and injuries of this nature, my eyes were shut to any other possibilities.

At work in my body were some nasty bacteria that had found their way in during the accident. I didn't realize how bad the infection was until I checked myself back into Royal Columbian Hospital on Labour Day, four months after the accident. Blood tests revealed that my leg was so full of infected fluid that there was concern it would burst under the pressure.

That second week of September, I underwent my fourth surgery, with a new surgeon, Dr. Darius Viskontas. He was the exact person I needed working on my case. He specialized in lower body reconstruction, and his skill and experience gave me the best chance for a positive outcome.

What happened to hope through all of this? The hope I had was lost, replaced by a major dose of realism. With that realism came a struggle, darkness, and questioning. It was proof positive that true hope has to have both an expectation and grounds for believing that expectation can become a reality.

Hopelessness is an essential foundation

How did I move from having my hopes dashed to finding new hope? I started by embracing hopelessness. Hopelessness served as the necessary bedrock on which I could start building again.

Once I had admitted my hopelessness, I could start to recognize the grounds for new hope. For me, it began with having a proper diagnosis. It took a while, but eventually the doctors and specialists determined the true nature of my condition and mapped out a pathway for moving forward.

Henri Nouwen observed, "Hope prevents us from clinging to what we have and frees us to move away from the safe place and enter unknown and fearful territory." As I descended into hopelessness, I made several other discoveries. I discovered the freedom to admit weakness, and I discovered new ideas for using my talents to help others. I realized that all kinds of people were willing to support me. I discovered fresh motivation based on the renewed plan for moving forward. And I discovered strength from God, who met me in my weakness.

There are three essential steps for discovering new hope.

1. Learn to read the warning signs of hope deprivation.

The better you are at reading the warning signs of hope deprivation, the quicker you'll recover when your hope is dashed. The signs I learned to read included being trapped by outdated expectations, seeing no pathway to get from where I was to where I wanted to be, losing the will to work for a better future, losing the ability to believe things would improve, and developing an aversion to risk.

Warning signs were plentiful in those early days of my recovery. My expectations were outdated, I didn't have a clear pathway, and the will to fight had drained out of me. I feared for the worst, and I wasn't sure I could handle any more pain and suffering. That wasn't the whole picture, but I needed to be aware of my loss of hope in order to start regaining it.

2. Fight for true hope.

You can't live for long without expectations for the future that are connected to a realistic pathway for getting there. If you have a future expectation and a pathway for getting there, you have the wings required to soar. Emily Dickinson put it this way: "Hope is

the thing with feathers that perches in the soul and sings the tune —
without the words — and never stops at all."

Renewed hope doesn't just happen. You need to fight for it by
exercising your faith muscle. Faith is all about believing in
something that you cannot see but are convinced by the evidence is
real. Try living for one minute without air. You don't see it, but it is
essential for life. True hope is "faith in the future tense," or, as
Jürgen Moltmann put it, "Hope is imagination placed in the
harness of faith."

3.   Find traction for renewed hope.

There are several ways to find traction when hope is lost and needs
to be reborn. Here are five of those ways:

- **Embrace the misery.**

William Shakespeare wrote, "The miserable have no other
medicine but only hope." Bertrand Russell added, "Extreme hopes
are born of extreme misery."

- **Start walking.**

You get traction by moving even when you don't feel like it. Barack
Obama advised, "If you go out and make some things happen, you
will fill the world with hope."

- **Move towards the light.**

Even if the light you see is extremely faint and distant, start moving
towards it, and let it grow stronger. Walter Scott said, "Hope is
brightest when it dawns from fears."

- **Do activities focused on others.**

Traction in hope happens when we help others, forgive the wrongs
done to us, say thanks, play, and are nice. Bruce Barton said,
"Before you give up hope, turn back and read the attacks that were
made upon Lincoln."

- **Take a leap of faith with the little bit of faith you have.**

Exercising the little bit of faith you have in God will lead to more
faith. The word "hope" is derived from the shorter word "hop,"

which can lead to "leap." Joan M. Erikson said, "To hope means to take a playful leap into the future—to dare to spring from firm ground—to play trustingly—to invest energy, laughter. And one good leap encourages another— On then with the dance."

A story of hope

I conclude this chapter with a story told by Nelson Mandela, who, when he was in Robben Island Prison, was inspired to hope during a visit from his daughter. The visit occurred shortly after his daughter Zeni married Prince Thumbumuzi. As a member of the Swazi royal family, she now had diplomatic privileges that allowed her to visit her father any time. She was able to meet with Mandela in an open room and brought along her newborn daughter. Mandela tells the story:

> I waited for them with some nervousness. It was a truly wondrous moment when they came into the room. I stood up, and when Zeni saw me, she practically tossed her tiny daughter to her husband and ran across the room to embrace me. I had not held my now-grown daughter virtually since she was about her own daughter's age.
>
> It was a dizzying experience, as though time had sped forward in a science fiction novel, to suddenly hug one's fully grown child. I then embraced my new son and he handed me my tiny granddaughter whom I did not let go of for the entire visit. To hold a newborn baby, so vulnerable and soft in my rough hands, hands that for too long had held only picks and shovels, was a profound joy. I don't think a man was ever happier to hold a baby than I was that day.
>
> The visit had a more official purpose and that was for me to choose a name for the child. It is a custom for the grandfather to select a name, and the one I had chosen was Zaziwe—which means "Hope."

The name had special meaning for me, for during all my years in prison hope never left me — and now it never would. I was convinced that this child would be a part of a new generation of South Africans for whom apartheid would be a distant memory — that was my dream.[2]

Nelson Mandela persevered day after day during his incredibly long prison sentence. More than once, he struggled to maintain hope, but he never gave up the fight. Eventually, he led his country to freedom and a new beginning because every time his hope was dashed, he adjusted, found new reason to hope and new grounds for believing, and pressed on.

Like Mandela, I aim to keep in my sights a better and brighter future.

Detour Reflections

❖ What inspires you to keep hope alive in your life?

❖ What about Nelson Mandela's story encourages you?

Chapter 3: Complaining

When your road ends abruptly, you need to complain. I used to see complaining as negative and something to avoid at all costs, but now I see it does have a place during recovery.

To complain means "to state one's displeasure or dissatisfaction" or "to state that one has pain or discomfort." The root of the word means "to lament." The word also has a medical meaning—what a patient does when telling the doctor where it hurts.[3]

Complaining is a natural and normal reaction to pain, and it helps the doctor to help you. One of the questions I heard multiple times after the accident and after every surgery was: "On a scale of one to ten, how is your pain?" The doctors and nurses wanted me to complain so they could give me the right dose of pain medicine. I didn't complain about that!

Legitimate complaining vents emotion, expresses reality, describes the facts, and keeps us grounded. Complaining only becomes unhealthy when it turns into whining and starts to negatively impact both the complainer and those around him.

What to do with long-term pain

If you are forced to endure emotional, physical, psychological, relational, or mental pain, how do you cope with it? How do you keep yourself from spiraling downward into a dark place of chronic complaining that turns toxic?

In the early days of coming to terms with my broken and pain-racked body, my complaints were frequent. The complaints persisted as each surgery ended, only to be followed by yet another painful surgery. The need to complain was undeniable. I was forced to wrestle with pain, swelling, exhaustion, and the continued loss of freedom and mobility.

How did I cope? I turned to history. I read the stories of people who had gone through extreme suffering but had learned to complain legitimately. One man who showed staying power and the kind of character qualities I wanted was Viktor E. Frankl. Frankl was a psychiatrist who spent the years from 1942 to 1945 as a prisoner in a German concentration camp. His book, *Man's Search for Meaning*, describes his experience in horrific detail, along with laying out a way to live in the worst circumstances. He quoted Nietzsche's words: "He who has a why to live for can bear with almost any how."

Viktor Frankl's three key ideas

To succeed in life, you need a future goal — a why or an aim. Frankl described those with a why as the strong ones, the ones able to bear the terrible how of their existence. Frankl wrote, "Woe to him who saw no more sense in his life, no aim, no purpose, and therefore no point in carrying on."

Frankl pointed out the difference between naive hope and true hope. He said the majority of the prisoners in the concentration camp lived with the naive hope that they would be home by Christmas. As Christmas drew near and there was no encouraging news, the prisoners lost courage and were overcome with disappointment and death. Those with true hope believed they would get out but did not hold to specific dates. They learned to find meaning in their day-to-day circumstances.

The three key ideas that Frankl taught were:

1. Life has meaning under all circumstances, even the most difficult ones.

2. Our main motivation for living is our will to find meaning in life.

3. We have freedom to find meaning in what we do and what we experience, or at least in the stand we take when faced with a situation of unchangeable suffering.[4]

What helped me apply these principles to my own life were these words of Frankl: "It does not really matter what we expect from life, but rather what does life expects from us." I had a choice during my prolonged time of adversity. I could either remain angry with God, life, the other driver, and other people or I could look for a reason to live, carry on, and add value to others. I chose to look for a deeper reason to live, and, because of that, I found a way to stay reasonably sane in spite of my challenging circumstances. It wasn't easy to stay focused on the bigger picture while feeling dissatisfied, but that decision gave me a handle to hold on to while walking in the darkness.

How to move from "Why?" to "What now?"

There is a time and place to ask, "Why?" Asking "Why?" helps us be real and honest about what we're experiencing during a loss and adversity. More than once I asked God why this accident had happened to me. When I first woke up, I found myself unusually calm and at peace, but as time wore on and the losses piled up, a deep complaint stirred within me .

Questioning why bad things happen is not abnormal. When we suffer loss or experience pain, we need to complain about our suffering and to find a way to vent our anger. The problem with asking "Why?" is that in time it stops serving a purpose and starts to take us in a downward direction.

How do we know when it's time to let go of our complaining? That's a great question and one that depends on our particular situation. I'm not sure when I made the shift exactly, but I do know that it took a great deal of reflection, outside intervention by skilled helpers, and a lot of soul-searching before I was finally able to do it.

If we want to grow through our "Why?" a better question we need to start asking is "What now?" Asking "What now?" sets the wheels in motion for turning complaining into contentment. Asking "What now?" calls us to dig deeper and find purpose in our pain and struggle. Asking "What now?" gets the focus off the blame game and onto solutions. It turns our focus outward instead of inward. It opens up new options and new opportunities for personal growth. Asking "What now?" starts the movement toward healing and wholeness.

Moving from "Why?" to "What now?"

What kept me stuck in an endless loop of asking "Why"? What kept me from moving on to "What now"? The list includes bitterness, lack of forgiveness, pain, shortsightedness, frustration, ignorance, and negativity. Here are the steps that are necessary if you want to move on.

1. **Step down.**

Moving to "What now?" starts with a deliberate choice to step down from continually asking "Why did this happen?" It may not feel right to stop questioning—pain, anger, frustration, and guilt are powerful forces trying to keep you stuck where you are—but it is the right thing to do if you want to truly live. Standing firm on the battlement of "Why?" makes your heart hard, keeps you acting as a victim, allows no room for forgiveness, and squelches the fresh thinking required to move forward into a renewed life.

2. **Step back.**

After you have stepped down, you need to step back and take a look at the options "What now?" can bring. Stepping back is taking stock of what you have to work with. It's about going up to the 30,000-foot level and looking around to see what your options are. It involves taking inventory of your talents, assets, and potential. Like stepping down, it's a choice—to believe that "Things will get better somehow."

3. Step into.

Once you have stepped down from asking "Why?" and stepped back to see your options, you will be ready to step into positive action. In the words of Mark Twain, "The secret of getting ahead is getting started." Stepping into is all about taking action to make "What's next?" a reality. Taking action leads to positive feelings you haven't experienced for some time and to the discovery of new meaning.

We often think that when we have recovered a positive attitude, then we will be able to take positive action. Actually, the reverse is true. Vaughan Quinn says, "The only way to get positive feelings about yourself is to take positive actions. Man does not live as he thinks, he thinks as he lives."

4. Step together.

Shortly after God created Adam, he said these words: "It is not good for the man to be alone."[5] We have a real need for traveling companions when times are good. However, our need for companionship and supportive friends increases tenfold when we go through hardship. "What now?" should not be asked in isolation. It requires the right friends, family, and support to be answered properly.

Detour Reflections

❖ What is the difference between legitimate complaining and unproductive whining?

❖ What structures (methods, tools, or practical aids) could you use to help facilitate healthy complaining?

Chapter 4: Now

Ralph Waldo Emerson said, "With the past, I have nothing to do; nor with the future. I live now." Two things keep us from living in the now — the past and the future. What we do with these two threats determines the quality of our lives.

When the world I knew was interrupted by the chaos and mess of the crash, it threw me into a tailspin. When the road ended, my mind avoided the present because it hurt. It was easier to dwell on the past, which looked so good looking back, or to fixate longingly on the future, when things would be "normal" again. I learned quickly, however, that *now* was the only reality I had. The past was in my memory, and the future was in my imagination. There is a time and a place to reflect on past memories and to dream of future possibilities, but that is only possible when our feet are firmly grounded in *now*. But I wondered, "How do I get there?"

It started when I separated fact from fiction.

Facts that anchored me in the *now*

1. Yesterday is not better than today, just different.

Fiction says, "Yesterday was better than today." Fact says, "Yesterday was different from today." Using the word "better" is all about comparing one thing with another. If you compare yesterday with today after a traumatic event, it doesn't help. It only keeps you stuck in your past since the past seems so much better.

The truth is that yesterday is different from today, not better or worse. Parts of yesterday might have been better, and parts might have been worse, but it doesn't matter. When I couldn't roll over in bed and had to be turned every two hours, it was best to be fully present with my immobility rather than to remember what I used to be able to do.

Edna Ferber warned, "Living in the past is a dull and lonely business; looking back strains the neck muscles, causing you to bump into people not going your way."

2. Yesterday I made a difference, and today I can as well.

We all want to contribute, to make the world a better place, to make a difference. But when I compared the quality and quantity of the differences I had been making before my road ended to the quality and quantity of the differences I was making afterward, I was miserable. It was disheartening to see what I was missing out on. I felt that the impact I was having had dropped significantly, and I didn't see the difference I was making now. I was like the person described in Alexander Graham Bell's words: "When one door closes, another door opens; but we so often look so long and so regretfully upon the closed door, that we do not see the ones which open for us."

I had no idea the difference I was making in people's lives while I was lying in that hospital room. My eyes were closed to present opportunities because they were glued to the past impact I had once had. I failed to see the opportunity I had right there and then to make a difference. I did not understand what Napoleon Hill had said: "Your big opportunity may be right where you are now."

3. When I stopped comparing tomorrow to yesterday, I could live in the present.

Fiction says, "What lies ahead pales in comparison to what I left behind." Fact says, "What lies ahead is in the future and needs to stay there. Now is where you need to live." The voice I heard inside my head said, "Life right now is terrible and will only get worse. If only you could go back to the life you once had. It was truly amazing!" That voice really messed me up.

What I learned was that I needed to be a student of today — to study it, learn from it, be fully present with it. I called it Trial University (TU), and recognizing that I was a student helped me stay present with what was right in front of me. I realized my previous life hadn't been perfect and the sooner I let go of that life, the sooner I could get to *now* and learn to deal with the pain and suffering. After all, as L. Thomas Holdcroft said, "The past is a guidepost, not a hitching post."

4. **Losing yesterday stole my confidence, but then I realized I could get it back.**

When my road ended, my confidence took a major hit. I felt insecure about what I'd be capable of doing in the future since I had lost my ability to work and didn't know when or if I would get that ability back. When you lose your confidence, your mind goes to the past (when you had confidence) and to the future (when you fear you won't have it).

What helped settle me down and live in the *now* was the realization that the method I had used to build up my confidence in the past would be the same method I could use in the future. It was true that my work had been put on hold. It was also true that some of my ability had been lost. However, it was also true that I could get my competence and confidence back through practice and hard work.

What living in the *now* gave me—and how I got there

I received a long list of assets and gifts when I began living in the *now*. I gained a heightened self-awareness. I developed an ability to grieve my losses—since I could be fully with the pain. I experienced less anxiety. I saw doors opening to help others. I discovered new ideas and new ways of seeing the world. I experienced unexpected joy and peace.

How did I get to *now*? I'd be lying if I said it was quick or easy, but there were some actions I took and some attitudes I embraced that made the journey to *now* possible. The experience will be different for everyone, but I believe many of these principles are universal.

It started with being aware of where I was and what I was going through—rather than being in denial or wishing I was somewhere else. I also had to let go of regrets and memories that were keeping me stuck. I had to learn to be OK with an unknown future (which was pretty hard for a control freak) and to exercise the little bit of faith I possessed. I had to be open to all of the sensory signals coming at me—sight, sound, touch, smell, and taste. I also readied myself to ask for help when needed and to be content to learn as much as I could along the way.

One dark day during my recovery, I came face to face with the realization that I was an emotional wreck. Instead of running from the raw emotions I was experiencing, I decided to stay present with them, and through that I eventually found peace. The peace came when I said with confidence, "I'm OK with not being OK."

Grabbing all the fruit you can

One of the phrases that describes how we should live in the *now* is the Latin phrase, *carpe diem*, which means "seize the day." *Carpe diem* comes from *carpe*, which means "pick, pluck, cull, gather, eat, enjoy, make use of," and *diem*, which means "day." In time, *carpe diem* came to mean the opposite of putting all your eggs in the future basket. Other ways to say it are "Grab today's fruit while it is ripe" and "If not now, then when?" (a Hebrew saying).[6] Henry David Thoreau put the idea this way: "I went into the woods because I wanted to live deliberately. I wanted to live deep and suck out all the marrow of life…to put to rout all that was not life; and not, when I came to die, discover that I had not lived."

A short time into my recovery, I came to realize I needed a major attitude adjustment. I was fluctuating between the past and the future, and it was keeping me from moving forward. As I gradually adjusted my perspective, the dark days of melancholy and hopelessness were replaced by the light of a new perspective. I was finally able to be fully attentive to and embrace what was going on in the moment (pain, people, and possibilities).

Three final thoughts on finding purpose in the *now*

1. Match expectations to reality.

A neat and tidy life is a fantasy. Life gets messy, pain happens, and loss is inevitable. Therefore, do not be surprised by suffering. If you expect your life to proceed smoothly, your unrealistic expectations will lead to even greater stress. When the road I was on ended, I was launched on a learning curve. I had to learn to live one day at a time and adjust my expectations to reality.

2. Allow yourself to be present with your pain.

Being present with your pain may hurt now, but avoiding or covering up pain will lead to even greater pain in the long run. Being with your pain does not answer all your questions or minimize the size of your challenge. It does lessen the possibility of anger taking root and your life being more miserable.

3. Act with love and kindness to all you meet.

No matter how bad it gets, your example and attitude can be a bright light to those around you. Showing love and kindness not only brightens the day of others but makes you feel just a little bit better as well. While being cared for by nurses, doctors, physiotherapists, and cleaning staff, I always made a point to treat them as I wanted to be treated. What came back to me was love and friendliness, which helped me get through what I was going through.

Detour Reflections

❖ In what way are you letting the past or the future interfere with your present living?

❖ What makes a day valuable to you?

Chapter 5: Choice

Between stimulus and response is a space. In that space is the freedom to choose our response. That choice has the potential to produce growth and happiness — or inertia and despair.[7]

When my somewhat predictable life was thrown into a state of chaos and pain, I struggled daily to make wise choices about how I would live. I felt as if I was driving down a highway in a Saskatchewan blizzard with limited visibility. All I had was the taillights of a Greyhound bus in front of me. On that bus were my faith that God would see me through, the friends and family members who walked with me, and the team of medical experts who were handling my case.

Choosing is an important part of everyday life, whether your road has just ended or not. According to a Duke University study, 40 percent of our decisions are habitual, decisions made without thinking.[8] The other 60 percent of our decisions require a conscious choice, made in that crucial space between stimulus and response.

The day I had a choice to make

One week after the accident, I was hit by a wave of unexpected trouble. Using a ceiling lift, the hospital staff were gingerly moving me from my bed to a wheelchair to give me a change of scenery. Since my right leg was broken in two places and my right arm in one, the only way to move me was to make use of this mechanical device. As the staff lifted my body out of bed, my right leg sprung a serious leak. The black liquid that poured out of it was unlike anything I had ever seen or smelled. It was black and ugly, a sure sign of infection. I was shocked and felt a darkening despair wash over me. Visiting us at the time was a former cattle buyer from the prairies, who said out loud: "That smells like a dead cow." It was, therefore, no surprise to learn that the bacteria that was infecting my leg, robinsoniella peoriensis, was a type usually found in manure pits. My exposed femur had picked it up off the highway.

The day after this happened, I underwent surgery to install a pump in my leg to drain the fluid. In addition to the pump, I received a diagnosis that put a major monkey wrench into what I had thought would be a speedy and uneventful recovery.

The robinsoniella peoriensis in my leg wasn't about to die without a fight—at the time, I had no idea how big a fight. Within two weeks, I had my third surgery—to remove the pump, put the leg in its proper position, and continue with the antibiotics necessary to kill the invisible enemy lurking inside my leg.

During those days, I was faced with a daily choice: Do I hope or do I despair?

Freedom to choose, freedom not to choose

When you are met with unexpected bad news, you are free to make one of two choices. You can choose to accept the bad news and hope for a better future, or you can choose to give up and believe hope is lost.

You are not free, however, to choose the consequences of your choice. It goes something like this: If you choose hope and see adversity as an opportunity for growth and change, your character will grow, and you will inspire others. If you choose to give up, quit looking for a greater purpose, stop reaching out for help, and give in to despair, you will be swallowed up by your own negativity and lose your way.

The choice to believe that I would somehow get through my current difficulties gave me traction to keep putting one foot in front of the other. I was devastated by the unfolding impacts of my accident and the changes that were being thrust upon me. However, somehow I found the inner strength to keep choosing to hope and to deal with each challenge as it came.

I made a number of choices:

- I chose to keep going even when I wanted to quit.
- I chose to believe things would get better even when they got worse.
- I chose to look for beauty around me and speak words of gratitude to others.
- I chose to minimize my whining and keep it to a necessary minimum.
- I chose to pray my way through pain and take God up on his offer of strength.
- I chose to trust that God knew what he was doing and would bring about some good despite all the trouble.
- I chose to fill my mind and imagination with stories that inspired hope.
- I chose to let go of the things I had lost and leave them behind.
- I chose to let go of end dates and unrealistic expectations.
- I chose to find little ways to make a difference in the lives of others.

Even though we have trouble in this world, we have the power to choose. An old proverb advises: "We cannot direct the wind, but we can adjust our sails."

A lesson from the sea turtle

On the Big Island of Hawaii, visitors occasionally encounter a bale of green sea turtles hovering on the ocean's edge. The perilous journey of the newborn turtles sheds some light on the power of choosing well.

The cycle of life for the turtle begins when the female crawls slowly onto shore sometime between May and August to dig a hole and lay her one hundred eggs. The turtle eggs incubate deep down in the sand for two months, and then the turtles hatch and emerge from the sand—but they only survive if they find their way safely to the ocean. The key to their survival is for them to follow the brightest horizon, which in a perfect world would lead them to the ocean. But the world is an imperfect place. Beaches once free from human development have been invaded by artificial light — from lamp poles, restaurants, homes, and condominiums. Artificial light can mean death to the young turtles if they confuse the artificial lights with the real thing and move in the wrong direction.

What's true for the newborn turtles can also be true for us. We sometimes choose the brighter artificial light instead of the true light because it arouses our curiosity and interest. All kinds of artificial lights exist which can take us in the wrong direction. When faced with a long recovery, I was surrounded by artificial lights. Distractions were everywhere, and they played on my emotions, attitudes, and actions. The artificial lights included chasing things outside my control and letting the annoying habits and attitudes of people get on my nerves. I worried about the future, spent too much time on technology and gadgets, and focused on results instead of the process of recovery. I kept conversations superficial and soft so I could avoid deeper dialogue. I stayed busy, only to find my time filled with activities void of meaning and purpose.

Guidelines for finding the right light to follow

There were three guiding principles I used to help me move in the right direction and find the life I was looking for.

1. Core values serve as a guide for life.

Because I had identified my core values before the accident, I had them to fall back on when I woke up. My list of values included connecting with God and family, making a difference, being real, and being a lifelong learner. With these values showing me the way, I dug myself out of a deep hole. They shone as lights in the darkness.

Shortly after Vicky had gone home to stay with her parents for a while in order to continue her recovery, I was joined in the next bed by a man who had lost part of his leg in a train accident. I instantly connected with him. I listened to his story, prayed for him through the curtain, and comforted him in his suffering. I felt alive in that moment as I made a difference in his life and helped him connect to the help God wanted to give him during his time of struggle.

2. Self-awareness gives insight necessary for change.

I lost track of the number of times I looked at my beaten and bruised body and said to myself, "What's going on with me? Am I the person I want to be right now? Is there anything I can correct or improve while I'm down here? Is it time for me to make some changes?"

It is natural—and necessary—to focus on "self-care" when you're in pain. What I learned, however, was that I needed to shift that natural self-focus, deepen my learning, and use the opportunity to adjust my character. In the hospital, I discovered nurses responded more quickly to my needs because I was kind and grateful, unlike the miserable, negative patient down the hall.

3. It is helpful to process hard news and loss with patience.

I found that the sooner I normalized bad news, the sooner I was prepared to deal with the aftermath of bad news. The earth is broken. Because of that, people mess up, evil happens, and mistakes are made. It is not easy to process hard news and live patiently when your days are slow and tedious, but it is possible. The good news is that, unlike sea turtles, who must operate on instinct, we have the ability to learn how to think, adapt, and change direction when we realize we're on the wrong path.

A final strategy for choosing wisely

When you learn to say "No," sometimes it opens up the door to saying "Yes." It isn't always obvious, but sometimes it is a lack of the ability to say "No" that holds people back. A "Yes" that flows out of a definite "No" can open doors to all kinds of new possibilities.

For example, because I said "No" to blaming God for the accident, I was able to more quickly accept the accident and see it as something God had allowed for a reason. I also said "No" to self-pity and the unending "Why?" question. Saying "No" opened up the door to saying "Yes" to good grief and living in the *now*.

I also said "No" to keeping quiet and not telling anyone my story because it hurt too much. That "No" allowed me to say "Yes" to the student nurse who wanted to interview me for a paper she was doing on the recovery process. My "Yes" ended up being an inspiration to her.

I said "No" to the need to see an end to my recovery—and "Yes" to the learning and deeper changes that took place while I was on the road to recovery. I said "No" to focusing only on what I had lost—so I could say "Yes" to focusing on listening, encouraging, processing, praying, supporting, and making a difference with my life.

Detour Reflections

❖ What do you need to say "No" to so you can say "Yes" to what really matters?

❖ How are the choices you are making today going to affect your future?

Part 2: The Detour

The detour is where the metal of character is forged. Detours have a way of slowing us down. They take us off the beaten track and onto a path that's rough and challenging. They require perseverance and patience.

When we are asked to take a detour, we usually don't have a choice. Because of that, we either make adjustments or we experience the downward spiral of a life that's out of control. Detours in life force us to go deep inside ourselves and learn to grow and change in order to survive.

The detour I was forced to traverse was the place where battles were fought, temptations were faced, and victories were won. On my detour, I attended some of the toughest classes Trial University (TU) had to offer. The curriculum included topics such as suffering, grief, waiting, the value of community, managing expectations, and persevering under fire.

Another way to describe the detour phase of a journey is to say it is "the messy middle." Healing occurs but intermittently and at its own pace. As you read Part 2, pay attention to how these themes intercept with your own journey, and remain open to the work you might need to do while on your detour.

Chapter 6: Endurance

Mary E. Pearson said, "Sometimes there's not a better way. Sometimes there's only the hard way." One of the qualities needed to travel the hard way is endurance. Endurance is defined as "the act, quality, or power of withstanding hardship or stress; the state or fact of persevering; continuing existence."[9] When the road I was on ended, the hardships and stress were overwhelming. I discovered very quickly that I needed to tap into endurance in order to rise to the new challenges I was facing.

Looking back, I realize that before the accident happened, I had had some practice in developing endurance. It came in the form of running and completing six marathons. Marathon racing is not for the faint of heart and requires ample endurance. To be honest, I'd rather run a marathon than suffer a near fatal motorcycle accident, but I wasn't given that choice. The need for endurance is most acute during the last six miles of a 26.2-mile marathon. The twenty-mile mark is usually where you have to start tapping into your inner strength in order to get to the finish line. At mile twenty, struggling with cramping calf muscles, an aching back, and an exhausted frame, I would ask myself, "Why am I doing this exactly? Am I crazy?" The answer always came back: "Because you can—and you will finish!" As I look back on those races, I wonder, "Could God have been preparing me for a different kind of marathon that would make 26.2 miles feel more like a five-kilometer training run in comparison?"

An Olympic tale of endurance

One of the ways I strengthened my endurance muscles was to read and listen to stories of endurance. The following story comes from the Olympic competition archives. It inspires me to endure every time I read it.

At 7:00 p.m. on October 20, 1968, a few thousand spectators remained in the Mexico City Olympic Stadium. It was cool and dark. The last of the exhausted marathon runners were being helped off to the first aid stations. More than an hour earlier, Mamo Wolde of Ethiopia — looking as fresh as when he had started the race — had crossed the finish line, winning the 26.2-mile event. As the remaining spectators prepared to leave, those sitting near the gates to the stadium suddenly heard the sound of sirens and police whistles.

All eyes turned to the gate. A lone figure, wearing number 36 and the colors of Tanzania, entered the stadium. His name was John Stephen Akhwari. He was the last man to finish the marathon. He had fallen during the race and injured his knee and ankle. Now, with his leg bloodied and bandaged, he grimaced with each hobbling step around the 400-meter track. The spectators rose and applauded him. After crossing the finish line, Akhwari slowly walked off the field. Later, a reporter asked Akhwari the question on everyone's mind: "Why did you continue to race after you were so badly injured?" He replied, "My country did not send me 7,000 miles to start the race. They sent me 7,000 miles to finish it!"[10]

Some of the many names for endurance

Let me put into words what endurance looks and feels like. As I endured sleepless nights, pain from surgery, the loss of what could have been, the endless waiting for the recovery to end, and the fear that I might lose my leg, I expressed the following phrases under my breath to help me take the next step.

- **Bite the bullet.**

Rudyard Kipling wrote: "Bite on the bullet, old man, and don't let them think you're afraid." The phrase "Bite the bullet" originated during a time in history when a wounded soldier was given a bullet to bite on to channel his reaction to intense pain. It was used before the invention of anesthesia in 1844. Thanks to William T.G. Morton[11] and other medical pioneers, I didn't have to bite the bullet when I had my surgeries. Instead, I had various forms of anesthesia, including a general, a spinal, a nerve block, and a failed epidural. I dreaded that rock hard surgery table and the prick of the needle going into my spine for the spinal especially—but when it was all over, I knew I had gone through yet another surgery with virtually no pain.

- **Take a deep breath.**

Taking a deep breath before something unpleasant can help prepare your mind and body for what is coming. While I had lost control of so many things, I still controlled my breathing. When my oxygen levels were low, I used an incentive spirometer that forced me to breathe deeply. When used repeatedly, this device increased the capacity of my lungs. Each breath contributed to my recovery and also flexed my endurance muscles.

- **Roll with the punches.**

This phrase originates in the boxing ring and paints a picture of resilience. "Rolling with the punches" describes a boxer who has the ability to bend slightly away from a punch, thus reducing its impact. This allows the boxer to bounce back and not suffer defeat at the first blow. Early on in my recovery, I was moved several times from one facility to another. One move in particular upset me greatly and felt like a punch in the gut. I had just been getting comfortable where I was, and I didn't want to move. Eventually, however, I changed my mind. I decided to roll with the punch of the transition. I realized I needed to keep moving so I wouldn't settle in a place of partial recovery.

- **Take it on the chin.**

This expression also comes from the boxing arena and paints a picture of someone who faces adversity courageously. The boxer "takes it on the chin" when he withstands punishment, perseveres against the odds, and bounces back from hardship. What I went through felt like being in a boxing ring. Some punches came out of nowhere, while others I saw coming. But I had to learn to take them all on the chin. I learned to endure each hit, look past the pain, and believe that I would survive to fight another day.

Shackleton as an endurance leader

One of the stories that stoked the fire of endurance and courage for me is the story of Ernest Shackleton's Trans-Antarctic Expedition. After their ship was trapped and then crushed in the ice, Shackleton led the other members of his team on a heroic journey across the ice on foot and then through perilous seas in lifeboats. Their ordeal lasted 634 days, in some of the harshest weather conditions on the planet. Under Shackleton's exceptional leadership, the crew maintained hope in circumstances that would have demoralized most other people.

There are many lessons that can be learned from Shackleton and his crew. One behavior that struck a chord with me was their ability to keep their eyes off their desperate situation and focused on tangible action. When they focused their energy on activities they could do together, they kept their minds off the horrific conditions all around them. For example, while trapped on the ice, Shackleton had his men march a little every day. Even though their progress was slow, it was better to keep moving than to sit down and "wait for the tardy northwesterly drift to take them out of this cruel waste of ice."[12]

When I compared my situation to Shackleton's predicament, I redefined what my future looked like and start moving slowly towards it. I learned how important it was to avoid sitting and waiting for the future to unfold: "The very act of doing something concrete creates a sense of momentum, and a series of small victories will lay the foundation for eventual success."[13]

Endurance needs the right perspective

Recovery is messy. You can have good days and bad days and days when you wonder if you're making any progress at all. This is all the more reason to keep the long view in mind and steel yourself for the journey, no matter how long it may be. One of the core beliefs that anchored my inner world was this: "This accident was an incident God allowed for a greater purpose I do not fully realize. It was no surprise to God and was filtered through his watchful eye. I surrender daily to his care and give him permission to use me as he sees fit."

Here are some steps to applying endurance:

- When the secure refuge you had counted on breaks apart and harsh circumstances force you to abandon ship, reset your destination and find a new target to focus on.
- When the race you are running gets harder than you ever imagined it could be, tap into your resourcefulness and believe you can endure beyond what you thought possible.
- When your situation seems impossible to live with, find a way to "keep moving."

Detour Reflections

❖ What metaphor for endurance resonates with you the most? How can it be applied to your life?

❖ What race are you in the middle of? Which step listed above will you choose to embrace while you run that race?

Chapter 7: Perspective

Oscar Wilde was speaking about the power of perspective when he reportedly said, "Two men looked through prison bars; one saw mud, one saw stars." When it feels like you're stuck in prison, you have a choice to make. You can either see mud and all that's terrible about your situation, or you can see stars and all that's possible in your situation.

My first couple of weeks in hospital felt like prison. I was awake but couldn't move. I was also in shock and dazed by what had transpired. I received tremendous support from family, friends, and hospital staff, but I felt that there were bars on my windows and there were no stars in sight.

Mud showed up in the form of a mangled body and an unknown road lying ahead. Three surgeries in ten days added more mud. One side effect of having three surgeries so close together was what the repeated general anesthetic did to my digestive system. I experienced serious constipation, accompanied by discomfort and pain. I was beyond frustrated and tried everything to get things moving. The nurse who finally helped me deal with this challenge was great. She was a little gruff, but I didn't care how friendly she was because she got the job done. I hated the bedpan and used it only because I had to, but the alternative was much worse.

A lesson on perspective

One of the ways I got through those early days was to see my situation from a different perspective. I decided to focus on what I had left, not on what I had lost. I searched high and low for things I could be grateful for—and soon found stars shining brightly through the bars of my prison cell.

I saw in my mind the helicopter crew landing on the highway and placing Vicky and me onto backboards for transport to the hospital seventy kilometers away. I saw Royal Columbian Hospital, the best trauma hospital in the province. I saw skilled surgeons keeping me alive and stitching me back together on the operating table. I saw nurses and a host of support staff changing my dressing and moving me carefully like clockwork when I couldn't move myself. I saw friends and family standing at our side to be present with Vicky and me as we healed. I saw in my mind and heart the thousands of people who didn't visit but who prayed for our recovery.

I had an incredible peace in those early days—a peace I can't fully explain. I very easily could have slid into a pit of despair, anger, and self-pity, but I didn't. Part of the reason I endured in those early days was the minute-by-minute choice I made to look for stars rather than mud.

Seeing things from God's perspective

There is a spiritual component to the prisons we find ourselves in. When I was lying in a hospital bed, I believed deep down that God would somehow use this event for a greater purpose. I believed that God had allowed the accident to happen and had not simply been caught napping that Saturday afternoon.

Because we live in a broken world, bad things do happen, and, as a consequence, we find ourselves in the midst of messy circumstances. But because of my faith in God and my belief that God had some purpose in my suffering, I was able to look for the stars and keep the mud in perspective. My trust in God wasn't automatically rock solid, but it increased over time as I kept reinforcing the perspective that what lay ahead for me was a purpose and a possibility, not a dead end.

Things are not always as they appear

Sometimes it pays to step back and consider a different point of view. If you jump to a conclusion too early, you miss seeing and hearing the additional information necessary to be able to gain a new perspective. Here is an apocryphal story that illustrates this very clearly:

Years ago in Scotland, the Clark family had a dream. Clark and his wife worked and saved, making plans for their nine children and themselves to travel to the United States. It had taken years, but they had finally saved enough money and had gotten passports and reservations for the whole family on a new ocean liner bound for the United States. The entire family was filled with anticipation and excitement about their new life. However, seven days before their departure, the youngest son was bitten by a dog. The doctor sewed up the boy but hung a yellow sheet on the Clark's front door indicating the possibility of rabies with a 14-day quarantine. The family's dreams were dashed. They would be unable to make the trip to America as they had planned. The father, filled with disappointment and anger, stomped down to the dock to watch the ship leave — without the Clark family. He shed tears of disappointment and cursed both his son and God for their misfortune. Five days later, the tragic news spread throughout Scotland — the mighty Titanic had sunk. The unsinkable ship had sunk, taking hundreds of lives with it. The Clark family was to have been on that ship, but because the son had been bitten by a dog, they were left behind. When Mr. Clark heard the news, he hugged his son and thanked him for saving the family. He thanked God for saving their lives and turning what he had felt was a tragedy into a blessing.[14]

Things are not always as they appear. Your perspective does matter. Events that on the surface look like tragedies can end up producing good fruit in our lives. On the other hand, the things that look like a blessing can end up tearing us apart.

There is no doubt our motorcycle accident was messy, painful, and difficult. However, I very quickly saw good coming from an event that was not what we would have described as good. The blessings that appeared included family closeness, deeper connections with friends, and a new appreciation for the things we had taken for granted. I also experienced opportunities to speak into people's lives, a greater appreciation for life, greater empathy for others who were suffering, and a deeper dependence on God.

The man and his goat

There were times during the early days of recovery when life seemed unbearable. I couldn't sleep, and I was constantly exhausted. The nights dragged on while the pain persisted despite the help of painkillers. During the day, I would attempt to read but would very quickly fall asleep or be unable to concentrate. I tried to write down my thoughts in my notebook, but after five short minutes had to quit. When the physiotherapists forced me to get out of bed and "move," it felt like all pain and no gain.

When life is a mess, it can be extremely challenging to maintain a healthy perspective. The man in the following story found life unbearable just as I did. The advice received from the rabbi has a powerful lesson for all of us.

There lived a man in Budapest who went to see his rabbi with the following complaint: "Life has become unbearable! I live a horrible life with eight other men in a one room apartment. What can I do?"

The rabbi answered with a simple solution: "Take your goat and bring him to live with you in the apartment." The man was dumbfounded and openly reacted to the idea, but the wise rabbi insisted, "Do as I say and come back to see me in a week."

The week went by, and the man returned looking more distraught than ever. "We cannot stand it," he told the rabbi. "The goat stinks, is destroying our furniture, and eats everything in sight!"

The rabbi gave his next set of instructions: "Now, go back home and put the goat back in his pen. Then, wait a week and come back and see me." The man obeyed.

A week later, the exuberant goat owner returned to the rabbi and exclaimed, "Life is beautiful! The nine of us haven't been happier now that the goat is gone. I can't thank you enough!"[15]

One of the ways I brought a goat into my hospital room was to look around at the people worse off than I was. It helped me appreciate how good I actually had it. I also read stories of people who had dealt with loss and adversity. Their stories made my situation pale in comparison. I also made a point to encourage and show gratitude to others, which worked to get the focus off myself and my problems and onto others.

Final thoughts

Changing your perspective and choosing to see stars, not mud is a daily choice. We have the power to make that choice, and when we do, everything changes. The words of Wayne Dyer are very fitting: "If you don't like the way something looks, change the way you look at it."

Detour Reflections

❖ What words would you use to describe your current perspective?

❖ Where in your life do you need a goat for a week? What might that experience teach you?

Chapter 8: Setbacks

Failure and setbacks can become a springboard for success. This belief isn't based solely on personal opinion but is backed up by a recent study. The study found that setbacks can create a breakthrough moment in our lives.[16]

Our accident was a major setback, and it was followed by a series of smaller setbacks. Setbacks happen for various reasons. Some are due to poor decision making — which was true in our case since the driver of the car that hit us pulled out in front of us when it was unsafe to do so. Other setbacks happen because of destructive choices. The reasons for other setbacks are not clear.

What matters most when a setback occurs is not why it happened but the way we respond. The reality is that two people can have the same setback and respond in completely different ways. Some people become mired in an endless pattern of self-pity and never get over their hurt or the damage done in their lives. Other people rise above their circumstances. Those who bounce back and recover from disappointment are called rebounders. Those who shrink back when met by disappointment are called recoilers.

Recoilers quit

Recoilers quit at the first sign of trouble. They give up the fight and splash around aimlessly in the mud of their affliction. They feel rattled because things didn't turn out the way they thought they would. They complain constantly and feel that the world is against them. They play the blame game and point the finger at others.

Recoilers rarely question their own judgment and assume they are always right. They overestimate their own abilities and lack the self-awareness to step back and see things from a different perspective. And yet they seem unable to solve their own problems.

Recoilers are surprised by failure and do not accept setbacks as a normal part of life. They fail to manage the flood of emotions that follows a devastating blow.

Rebounders don't

Rebounders are very different from recoilers because they learn from setbacks and failures. They "know how to solve problems and overcome setbacks, often because they've done it before…they tend to react with calm determination, and even a sense of humor, when something goes wrong. They'd rather solve problems than complain about them or blame someone else."[17]

Failure, to a rebounder, comes as no surprise but is seen as a normal part of life. Rebounders manage emotional fallout with honesty, self-reflection, and a decision to process the emotions they are experiencing. They are action oriented and respond by getting back up when knocked down. They have a growth mindset, embrace new ideas, let go of broken dreams, and throw away outdated thinking.

Rebounders have also learned to live with discomfort. They know that harsh conditions may actually be the pathway forward. They don't demand quick fixes but are patient and allow time to heal and recover. Learning to actively wait tilts the odds of a breakthrough in their favor. It was the ability to rebound rather than recoil that enabled Ernest Shackleton and his crew to survive after their ship was crushed in the ice of the frigid Antarctic.

Rebounders possess passion, but passion alone isn't enough. They also need an inner drive and a quality called resilience

My story of rebounding

Shortly after the accident, I accepted the road I was on as the one God had chosen for me to travel. Yes, my life changed dramatically after the accident. One of the most glaring changes was that even though my wife and I had enjoyed motorcycle riding for many years, we realized very quickly that we would need to give it up. As hard as that was to lay down, having the belief that we would rebound and find something else we loved moved us forward.

After the crash, I experienced a whole gamut of emotions. Instead of recoiling from the very strong painful emotions, I embraced the emotional roller coaster I had been thrown onto. I chose to accept and work through emotions such as uneasiness, worry, fear, isolation, defeat, impatience, and frustration. The upside was I could also embrace moments of joy, gratitude, relief, tranquility, and the warmth of being loved and cared for.

There were days when I didn't want to get out of bed and work with the smiling physiotherapists who began coming to my room right after surgery. But I chose to act as a rebounder instead of a recoiler. I welcomed these medical professionals as partners who inflicted pain not to be mean but to keep me from staying down any longer than I had to. If I recoiled one day, I regrouped and rebounded the next.

As a rebounder, I kept my eyes and ears open in order to learn from the people around me. When I kept my mind active, even when I was in pain, it helped me experience small breakthroughs. It is hard to put into words the peace I felt as I made the uphill climb, experienced setbacks, but continued to climb, never giving in to doubt, discouragement, or fear.

Each of us has the power to choose how to handle setbacks. We can either bury our head in the sand and hope things change or lean into the storm, adjust, and grow stronger. Leaning into the storms of life results in personal growth and breakthroughs we will not experience if we recoil from them.

Resilience: bouncing back after a setback

Resilience comes from an old Latin word meaning "to spring back" or "rebound." It is defined as the "ability to recover readily from illness, depression, adversity, or the like; buoyancy."[18]

In his book *Grit in the Craw,* Robert Luckadoo tells how he learned to fly an airplane. He practiced the takeoff and landing hundreds of times with his instructor present. But the time came to go it alone. The task was to get his plane, a Cessna 152, up in the air, go for a short flight, and land the plane on the first third of the runway. As he approached the landing, he repeated to himself, "You can do this! I know you can." With fear and trembling, he brought the Cessna in and nailed the landing. Reflecting on his first solo flight, he said:

> Learning to fly was something I'd always wanted to do. It was so important to me, that I was willing to go through all the necessary trials and tribulations to make it a reality. Going to the airport week in and week out and endlessly practicing takeoffs and landings took a tremendous amount of resilience. Until the day I was ready to solo, it was all about making mistakes and bouncing back from them. Making mistakes over and over and bouncing back over and over. And finally it all paid off. My first solo flight was in the books.[19]

Resilience and recovery

Resilience during recovery is critical. I worked for days and weeks to build up strength in my legs and flexibility in my knee and ankle, pushing through the pain and discomfort in order to get moving again. Then wham! I was hit by the setback of another surgery. I wondered in those moments, "Why bother doing all this work if I have to start all over again?"

Looking back on the many times I had to bounce back, I realized how important the work I had already done to build a stronger base helped me each time I faced a setback. Bouncing back after each setback prevented me from experiencing overwhelming discouragement and prepared me for the next battle I would face. Each series of steps in the recovery journey was like going on a practice flight that prepared me for the solo flight I would eventually take.

Resilience had a reward. It built muscle in my leg that I could use even after it was disturbed by another surgery. The strength I brought to the operating table each time was not completely lost. The health and optimism I gained during my practice flights was what I built on after each setback.

What was true in my physical recovery was also true in my mental, spiritual, and emotional recovery. Getting up after each fall made me stronger and more determined to keep pushing forward.

Final thought

Calvin Coolidge said, "Press on. Nothing in the world can take the place of persistence. Talent will not. Unrewarded genius is almost a proverb. Education will not. The world is full of educated derelicts. Persistence and determination alone are important." Persistence is the quality needed to get up each time you fall until you arrive at your destination.

Detour Reflections

❖ What changes in your life have put you back into transition and have felt like two steps backwards?

❖ What have you done in the past to help you get through future setbacks successfully?

Chapter 9: Adversity

Adversity is defined as "adverse or unfavorable fortune or fate; a condition marked by misfortune, calamity, or distress" and "an adverse or unfortunate event or circumstance."[20] When I woke up after the accident, misfortune, calamity, and distress were my reality. The accident was my misfortune, and calamity and distress followed – in the form of surgeries, infection, pain, and loss.

The intensity of adversity varies greatly. For some, it's relatively light and short-lived while for others, it's extreme and long-term. For me, it was like sailing through a violent storm, with highs and lows, joys and sorrows, improvements and setbacks. Every time I moved three steps forward, it felt like I then took two steps back.

How you respond to adversity changes everything

When I asked the doctors when I'd be healed, they gave vague answers because they didn't know how long the recovery would take. When I asked the doctors when I'd run again, they said, "It's hard to tell." In my mind, I saw myself back to work in three months and running races in six. I was determined to beat adversity into submission!

But my recovery was moving much more slowly than I thought it would. I was better prepared for what had hit me than I thought I would have been, but I don't think anyone could ever be fully prepared for a calamity as severe as the one that had hit me. I had never experienced that level of pain before. I had never felt so out of control as I did during the early days of my recovery. Initially, I felt overwhelmed. However, as I shortened my focus from "one day at a time" to "one minute at a time," I began to inch my way forward.

DETOUR

Three steps to adversity's dance

A metaphor I used to describe my adversity was to say it was something I was learning to dance with. To "dance with adversity" meant to reject the temptation to fight or flee and instead to accept, embrace, and deal with the misfortune I had experienced. I discovered that there were three steps to this dance.

1. Believe that God's purpose will prevail amidst difficulty and that good can come from it.

There is a Bible verse that is often misused: "And we know that God causes everything to work together for the good of those who love God and are called according to his purpose for them."[21] Properly understood, it is a promise to those who love God and choose to embrace his way of living—encouraging them to join in adversity's dance.

2. Learn to embrace adversity and not eliminate it prematurely.

There was another piece of instruction in the Bible that I found annoying, but that in the end provided part of the foundation on which I could rebuild my life: "Consider it a sheer gift, friends, when tests and challenges come at you from all sides. You know that under pressure, your faith-life is forced into the open and shows its true colors. So don't try to get out of anything prematurely. Let it do its work so you become mature and well-developed, not deficient in any way."[22]

3. Listen to the stories of others who have mastered adversity's dance.

Aimee Mullins inspired me to dance during my distress. She broke a record at the Paralympic Games in 1996 in spite of being born without shinbones. She described adversity not as something to be overcome but as something to be danced with: "There's a partnership between perceived deficiencies and our creative ability so it's not about sweeping under the rug the challenges but finding the opportunity wrapped in the adversity…Perhaps if we see adversity as natural, consistent and useful, we're less burdened by the presence of it."[23]

Michelangelo saw the big picture

In 1507, Michelangelo was commissioned by Pope Julius II to paint the ceiling of the Sistine Chapel. It was an honor to be asked, but he didn't jump into the project without stepping back first. He labored for months over hundreds of sketches, analyzing multitudes of colors and themes, before ever dipping his brush into the paint. Finally, he put up his scaffolding and started the work in 1508. The painstaking work of painting while lying on his back was finally completed in 1512.

One day, the story goes, Michelangelo was painting in an obscure corner of the Chapel when his frustration boiled over. He was so frustrated he painted over his work and started over. One of the workers in the Chapel said to Michelangelo when he saw what he had done, "Why worry over something nobody will ever see?" The great Michelangelo said, "I will know." Michelangelo had the big picture in mind. The big picture inspired him to endure, to keep going forward until his vision became a reality.

On another occasion, the Italian sculptor Agostino d'Antonio worked diligently on a large piece of marble. Finally, after much effort, he quit in disgust, saying, "I can do nothing with this!" Other sculptors tackled the piece of marble but also gave up—until Michelangelo. When Michelangelo saw the unfinished statue, he studied it for a while, mapped out a plan, and began to work. Four years later, the world laid eyes on one of the greatest pieces ever sculpted by Michelangelo—"David." The statue, started in 1501 and completed in 1504, stood fourteen feet, three inches tall and was placed outside the Palazzo Vecchio.

Borglum saw the big picture

Gutzon Borglum was the sculptor who pictured and chipped away for years to carve four faces out of the granite of Mount Rushmore. Like Michelangelo before him, Borglum saw the big picture long before he blasted away the first chunk of stone. Borglum had a vision of what he wanted to achieve before he started the tedious process of creating detailed likenesses of George Washington, Abraham Lincoln, Theodore Roosevelt, and Thomas Jefferson.

President Coolidge dedicated the carving as Borglum began work in 1927, but the faces would not be finished for another fourteen years. Unfortunately, Borglum died in March 1941, and his son Lincoln completed the project, which has now been admired by several generations. Was it a tragedy that Gutzon never saw the finished work? But he most certainly did see it! He saw it in his imagination in such vivid detail that it inspired both himself and his son to work tirelessly until it was completed.

When I saw the big picture about my accident, I settled down for the long haul. As part of the big picture, I saw a few things more clearly. I saw improved character taking shape in my own life. I saw friends, family, and onlookers rethinking what really matters. I saw through the eyes of faith the reward I would receive if I remained faithful to God's calling through my difficult circumstances. I saw how important my example could be for others.

No silver bullet

There is an old Eastern proverb that says, "The fox has many tricks, but the porcupine has one big trick." This applies perfectly to the dance with adversity. There is no silver bullet, no one solution we can use to deal once and for all with adversity. Adversity's dance requires agility, a variety of steps, creativity, and alertness.

Dr. Norman E. Rosenthal served as a clinical professor of psychiatry at Georgetown Medical School and learned seven tricks that helped people to dance with their adversity. I used these tricks in my own dance with adversity.[24]

1. **Accept the fact that adversity has occurred.**

I learned to pray the Serenity Prayer, which includes these powerful words: "Living one day at a time; enjoying one moment at a time; accepting hardships as the pathway to peace..."

2. **Proportion your response according to the nature and severity of the adversity.**

The response required after my accident was multi-faceted and constantly changing as new challenges and complications showed up. What was required of me after the accident was much different from what was required of me the time I drove my car into a mailbox and dented the hood.

3. **Analyze the situation.**

A trick I learned early on was to not panic but to engage my left brain immediately. I learned to think through the situation before drawing a conclusion.

4. **Regulate your physical and emotional state.**

As well as I was able, I used nighttime for sleeping, daytime for being awake, and mealtimes for eating. I exercised discipline in order to focus on positive and uplifting thoughts, as well as engaging in productive activity.

5. **Reach out for help.**

I valued the visits, support, and conversations I had with family, friends, and the professionals who worked with me. I reached out to strangers, who ended up becoming a readymade support group when no one I knew was there to talk to.

6. **Turn your predicament into a story.**

Telling my story helped me to navigate and process what I was going through. I ended up telling my story to anyone who would listen. I tried not to annoy people, but usually telling my story ended up helping us both, as long as I approached the conversation with self-awareness.

7. Reframe the adversity.

I regularly stood back in my imagination and looked at my life from a different perspective. This offered me a new way to see my calamity, which helped me gain new insights and handle the distress.

Final thoughts

Uplifting and inspiring words helped to hold me up and keep me strong during the darkest days. Even if I didn't fully believe these words when I read them, they eventually sunk in and shaped my life. Here are just a few of those wise sayings:
- "All sunshine makes the desert." – Arabian proverb
- "Fractures well cured make us more strong." – Ralph Waldo Emerson
- "Adversity is the mother of progress." – Mahatma Gandhi
- "The gem cannot be polished without friction, nor man be perfected without trials." – Danish proverb
- "Obstacles are great incentives." – Jules Michelet
- "Problems are only opportunities in work clothes." – Henry J. Kaiser

Detour Reflections

❖ What does "embracing adversity" mean for you?

❖ What would have to change to make "dancing with adversity" your perspective of choice?

Chapter 10: Emotions

To experience emotion is to have "energy in motion." The word emotion comes from an Old French word meaning "to excite" and from a Latin word meaning "to disturb" or "to move."[25]

When a road ends, when events and circumstances change the smooth road of our former reality into the bumps and dips of uncharted territory, an emotional ride begins. We are disturbed, excited, and moved to respond. The way we deal with this "energy in motion" makes all the difference. The more prepared we are for such experiences, the better.

Four parts to the emotional puzzle

When the road I was on ended, I was forced to navigate and manage many different emotions. It was a roller coaster ride unmatched by anything I had experienced to that point in my life. I realized rather quickly that if I was to survive, stay hopeful, and dance with the emotional backlash, I had to make major adjustments. I had to take a crash course on how to deal with emotions and how they could contribute to my growth, not get in the way of it.

In the early days of my recovery, I identified four parts to the emotional puzzle that needed my attention. These four components helped me see emotions as a friend, not an unwelcome guest. I needed emotional self-awareness, the ability to dance with my emotions, emotional self-mastery, and the ability to cry deeply.

1.   Emotional self-awareness

Tao Te Ching said, "Knowing others is intelligence; knowing yourself is true wisdom." For me, emotional self-awareness was the doorway into a whole inner world. Without emotional self-awareness, I would have stayed stuck after my traumatic accident and the subsequent prolonged chaos. The words of Jean de La Fontaine reinforced my need for self-awareness: "He who knows the universe and does not know himself knows nothing."

What is emotional self-awareness? It is "the ability to recognize your feelings, to differentiate between them, to know why you are feeling these feelings, and to recognize the impact your feelings have on others around you."[26] It is about increasing your capacity to explore and understand what is happening to you so you can respond appropriately.

When we lack self-awareness, we are more likely to become sarcastic, disrespectful, frustrated, and angry. When I saw my emotional health struggling, it gave me the information I needed to reach out for more help. Had I not seen the emotional pain I was experiencing, I'm not sure I would have been so open to seek and receive help. During the months of therapy, I can attest to the fact that I made progress as I gained a greater understanding of what exactly was going on. When it comes to emotional healing, it is impossible to treat what you are unaware of.

There is a proverb that says, "When you are looking in the mirror, you are looking at the problem. But remember you are also looking at the solution."

2. Dancing with emotions

Emotional self-awareness is a great starting point but only part of the process. The puzzle piece that goes with awareness is the willingness to dance with what we are experiencing emotionally. Putting a name to the emotion we are experiencing is part of that dance, and there are many partners.

My list of emotional partners included guilt, disappointment, peace, fear, tension, surprise, sorrow, serenity, shock, sentimentality, sadness, resentment, pity, outrage, misery, loneliness, love, joy, homesickness, humiliation, grief, grumpiness, envy, and anger. My emotional dance felt a little like driving in a Saskatchewan snowstorm. My eyes were open, and I was staring out through the windshield, but all I could see were big white flakes and poorly marked lines to the right and left. I was afraid that at any minute I could miss a corner and find myself in the ditch or on the other side of the road in oncoming traffic.

I have never been much of a dance partner, but I do understand the theory. One thing I know from the little bit of dancing I have done is that it is necessary to find a balance between analyzing my movements and feeling the rhythm of the music, which will allow me to enter into the experience I am having with my partner. The dancing metaphor breaks down a little because physical dancing is usually a pleasurable experience while dancing with emotion during recovery can have some significant elements of pain.

I learned to be conscious of the way I felt and to put those feelings into words. I would say to myself, "I feel this way because..." Identifying the trigger to the emotion helped me to dance with the emotion.

I didn't always dance with emotion alone either. With trusted friends, I told my story and found support and strength while dancing with emotion. Vulnerability hasn't always been easy for me, but I learned how important it was to the healing process. Proverbs 11:14 (MSG) advises, "Without good direction, people lose their way; the more wise counsel you follow, the better your chances."

3. Emotional self-mastery

Following on the heels of having emotional self-awareness and being able to dance with emotions is the need for self-mastery. Self-mastery is the ability to withstand the emotional storms that blow into our lives and is the opposite of becoming (to borrow a phrase from Hamlet) "passion's slave." If our passions run our lives, we are taken out of the driver's seat and left to blow in the winds of change. The goal with emotion is to find a balance between the extremes of emotional suppression and emotional excess. A life without passion would be a dull, gray wasteland of numbness. Emotional self-mastery works at finding emotional balance.

According to Aristotle, it involves appropriate feelings proportionate to the circumstance.

One emotion I dealt with frequently was sadness. Sadness hit me because of my losses, disappointments, and pain. My journey with sadness started with seeing it (self-awareness) and learning to embrace it (dancing with it), but then moved on to the point where I was able to let it ebb and flow within a range that would move me through it rather than leave me stuck in it (self-mastery).

Sadness wasn't negative—it just was. It was neutral, and it taught me something about myself. It became a messenger that told me there was work I needed to attend to. Sadness helped me come to terms with what I had lost and forced me to reduce my activities so I could focus on my emotional healing. Sadness put me into a "reflective retreat" mode so I could mourn, reflect, and process my grief.

Self-mastery relates to the whole spectrum of emotional reality. It calls us to respond with our whole being.

4. Valuing deep crying

Built into our beings is a physical mechanism intended to bring relief and inner healing. This mechanism scares a lot of people and is often avoided like the plague. The mechanism is the tears that flow from deep within. Crying is often misunderstood and underappreciated. We are born to cry. Tears exist to make us well. Deep crying relieves the pain and stress we feel inside and is a critical part of the journey of grief. Victor Hugo warned, "Those who do not weep, do not see."

Tears were a close companion during my recovery. They weren't always welcomed, but they were critical to keep me moving forward in my recovery. Deep crying is different from superficial tears. Deep crying heals the soul and unlocks the door to the inner journey to wholeness.

Five months into my recovery, I hit the skids emotionally and physically. I had an unplanned emergency surgery to deal with the infection that was still active deep inside my leg. It felt as if I could hear the screeching of brakes all over again, bringing my life to a dead stop. My life was out of control, and the road ahead had suddenly become longer and rockier. That month of September was a dark time. I was ready to snap at the next person who asked me how I was doing. I was angry and confused, a mess.

But during that month, something unexpected happened. I was hit by two experiences of deep crying. These crying sessions surprised me, but they helped me move forward in my inner healing. One deep crying session came while I was in my hospital room surrounded by Vicky and two of our closest friends. The crying hurt my gut, but it started to heal my soul. It was what I needed to let the grief out. The other deep crying session came just a couple of days later when a good friend sat by my bed and gave me the space to let another river of deep tears come pouring from deep within my soul.

During those deep crying sessions, my grief, anger, frustration, pain, and sorrow found a release, like the opening of a relief valve. Had someone offered the Kleenex box too soon, those healing tears might have been cut off prematurely.

Final thoughts

The emotional well is deep, and in all honesty I have barely scratched the surface. Every part of me was impacted when the road ended. The emotional highs and lows were extreme. I celebrated a win when I took my first few steps while holding onto the parallel bars under the supervision of my physiotherapist. I was overwhelmed with fear when I read my CRP score (CRP stands for C-reactive protein and measures infection levels in the blood). I was afraid I would end up losing my leg in spite of all the hard work that had been done.

One truth that became clear to me when I was faced with the emotional side of recovery was the preparation I had unknowingly made for this challenge. Thankfully, for many years I had been practicing emotional self-awareness, dancing with emotion, self-mastery, and healthy crying.

Detour Reflections

❖ What emotional puzzle piece do you do well? Where do you need to practice?

❖ What do you do when sadness becomes inappropriate and you find yourself slipping into unhealthy depression?

Chapter 11: Suffering

Once there was a man who found the cocoon of a caterpillar. As he stared at it, he noticed a small opening starting to form. He watched the budding butterfly for hours as it struggled to force its body through the little hole. All of a sudden, the struggle stopped and it looked as if the butterfly had gotten as far as it could on its own.

The man sprang into action and decided to help the butterfly. He grabbed a pair of scissors and started to snip the cocoon off the struggling body. To his delight, the butterfly emerged into the open air — but with a swollen body and small, shriveled wings. The man continued to watch the butterfly, waiting for it to spread its wings and lift off, soaring into the air. Instead, nothing happened. The butterfly spent the rest of its life crawling around on its belly with a swollen body and shriveled wings. It never did learn to fly.

In his desire to help the butterfly, what the man had done was to short-circuit the process required for the butterfly to be ready for flight. The butterfly's struggle to push itself out of the cocoon is nature's way of forcing fluid from the body into the wings. It is a necessary but solitary journey involving pain and adversity.

The place suffering has in our lives

Suffering has a similar place in our lives even when every bone in our body wishes there was another road to travel. Without suffering, we become soft and untested. We become unable to handle bad news and end up living selfish, shallow lives. If suffering and hardship are not part of our experience, our character will never fully develop, and we will fail to take risks for fear we will fall and hurt ourselves. Without our own suffering, we will be disconnected from the struggles of others.

Suffering creates the fertile soil from which new life can spring. A tree may provide shade for the weary traveler, but its roots didn't grow deep during calm weather but during times of drought and strong winds. Suffering helps us to develop a grateful heart and a persevering spirit. Suffering forces us to adjust to a new perspective and a new plan we didn't see before the test came

The pathway to peace

I learned a lot about suffering when it became not just a concept but a lived experience. Another word I came to equate with suffering was hardship. A prayer that I used often to put into words what I needed to say to God was the Serenity Prayer written by Reinhold Niebuhr. One line in particular stood out to me: "Accepting hardship as a pathway to peace." This particular line didn't make much sense when I first read it. How was it possible to accept hardship and end up with more peace? I thought it must be a misprint. But, as I reflected on my experience and took a deeper look, I saw the hope buried in those words. Here is the entire Serenity Prayer so you can see that phrase in context:

God, give me grace to accept with serenity
the things that cannot be changed,
Courage to change the things
which should be changed,
and the Wisdom to distinguish
the one from the other.
Living one day at a time,
Enjoying one moment at a time,
Accepting hardship as a pathway to peace,
Taking, as Jesus did,
This sinful world as it is,
Not as I would have it,
Trusting that You will make all things right,
If I surrender to Your will,
So that I may be reasonably happy in this life,
And supremely happy with You forever in the next.
Amen.[27]

What was it that resonated when I read the phrase "accepting hardship as a pathway to peace"? It took me back to the definition of true hope—"an expectation with a pathway to achieve it." For me, true hope during my season of suffering was the belief that no matter how hard the road became, peace would be found if I accepted hardship and suffering as part of the journey. In contrast, I realized that if I fought the suffering and labeled it unfair and unwelcome, I would remain stuck and miss out on the peace that was possible.

Hardship alone did not result in peace. I knew that because I watched others around me grow bitter and angry as they fought against their suffering. The key was to accept what had come, and in that acceptance I could see the door to peace open for me.

My natural tendency had been to look in all the wrong places for peace. I would say, "If I can just solve my problems, eliminate my hardship, lower my anxiety, reduce my stressors, get control back, or manage these difficult people, I will have peace." The problem with that approach was that in every case, peace depended on my circumstances getting better. That just wasn't happening.

If our circumstances don't improve quickly or if they never improve at all, do we then have to settle for "no peace" and perpetual misery? Not according to the words of this prayer—and not according to what I experienced. I learned firsthand that true peace was an "inside job," the by-product of the choice I had made to accept what was happening rather than fight against it.

Five shocking truths about pain

Pain might not be the enemy we make it out to be. At certain times, pain can actually be our friend and ally. Pain can be a traveling companion that serves as a catalyst for character growth and positive change. Robert Browning Hamilton's poem confirms that:

I walked a mile with Pleasure;
She chatted all the way;
But left me none the wiser,

73

For all she had to say.
I walked a mile with Sorrow;
And ne'er a word said she;
But, oh! The things I learned from her,
When Sorrow walked with me.[28]

When I was tempted to accuse God of messing up and letting pain happen for no good reason, I decided to challenge that premise. I reconsidered the potential value of pain and suffering in my life and eventually came to see its purpose and potential good. Some of our pain is the result of sin and a broken world, but not all of it.

1. Pain is a gift.

Without pain, we would have no warning signal that something is wrong. For example, people with leprosy have pain sensors that fail to function. The result is lost fingers due to hot stoves and bed sores due to the failure to roll over while sleeping. "Dr. Paul Brand came to appreciate pain by living among people with leprosy. It was he who discovered that leprosy patients suffer for the simple reason that they have a defective pain system."[29]

Some of the worst pain I endured was during the six months of new bone growth. I had a bone transporter sticking out of my leg, facilitating new femur growth inside my leg. One morning after a challenging night, I wrote this in my journal, "It was a tough night with pain—a burning tightness in my leg. I rubbed it and got some relief, but my leg feels enflamed with life as the new growth takes place. Does growth have to hurt so much? I guess it does, as it deals with the obstacles of muscle fibres and scar tissue and cuts a path down the inside of my leg." I grew weary and frustrated with the pain, but saw it ultimately as a gift that gave me a renewed leg.

2. Ninety-nine percent of all pain is short-term and correctable.

When pain serves as a warning signal that something is wrong and needs corrective action, it is truly our friend. According to Dr. Brand, many of the short-term pains we experience in the course of living indicate correctable situations that call for medication, rest, or a change in our lifestyle. The pain inflicted by my physiotherapists was in this category. It was not enjoyable, but I learned to see it in its proper perspective. I knew that pain was required to give me greater flexibility and break through the resistance built up due to the surgeries and the repair process.

When the physiotherapists leaned on my leg with all their weight and bent my knee as far as it could go, my eyes filled up with tears, and I would long for the treatments to end. What I learned, however, was that the pain was temporary and that it was the only way to greater healing.

3. Pain makes normal life possible.

If you are a healthy, functioning human being, pain cells in your body are at work all day long. They tell you when to go to the bathroom, when to loosen your grip on the rake, when to blink, and when to roll over in bed. Without pain, we would lead lives of paranoia, defenseless against unfelt dangers.

When the bone transporter did its painful work (I describe that process in the chapter on perseverance), it paved the way for a life that was closer to "normal" than would have been possible otherwise. I came within a hair's breadth of losing my leg, which would have taken my journey in a whole different direction. The painful experience of growing bone made something closer to normal possible.

4. Pain increases our ability to experience joy and pleasure.

When we experience pain, it has a way of turning up the volume on our "pleasure" sensors. After each major surgery, I would wake up eager to push the morphine pump. The other pleasure I would ask for was for the nurse to give me a sip of ice cold water, which felt so refreshing after all I had just gone through.

One of the ways I found pleasure in the midst of pain was to go for rides on my red scooter. I had my first ride shortly after the bone transporter was installed, which brought with it constant pain and discomfort. While on the scooter, I was in pain, but I found the

75

flowers more attractive and the conversations with my neighbors more stimulating. I enjoyed movies with compelling characters (such as *Batman* and *Men in Black*), listened to music, and revisited a buried talent of playing the piano.

5. Because the world is broken, not all pain is good.

There is a bigger reality at play here on this planet regarding pain. In some cases, pain is a consequence of evil deeds done by some people to other people. Certain pain is the result of God's creation having been marred by what is called "the fall of humanity." The reality of a broken world is hard to escape, and it does explain some of the pain we experience.

C.K. Chesterton described it this way: "According to Christianity, in making it [the world], He [God] set it free. God had written, not so much a poem, but rather a play; a play he had planned as perfect, but which had necessarily been left to human actors and stage-managers, who had since made a great mess of it." [30] Our accident was the result of human error and was not "good," and it produced pain.

Final thoughts

Suffering will be with us for as long as we live out our time here on this earth. If we accept the hardships that come into our life regardless of the source, we put ourselves on the path where deeper growth and meaning can be found. To fight pain as foreign and an unwelcome guest will lead to even more suffering, not less. Fierce pain can have a refining purpose in our lives, but it is not something that I recommend people go looking for.

Detour Reflections

❖ How does accepting hardship put you on the path towards peace?

❖ When in your life has pain been your friend?

Chapter 12: Grief

Grief is "keen mental suffering or distress over affliction or loss; sharp sorrow; painful regret."[31] Grief is not a "one size fits all" kind of thing, but it is a common experience of those who have suffered different types of losses. I grieved intermittently after the road ended. My grief didn't come in one continuous flow but was staggered and unpredictable. It came in waves, broken up by new experiences of loss. The affliction I experienced touched every corner of my life—mental, physical, spiritual, and emotional.

But my experience of grief was not entirely negative. The words of Leo Tolstoy rang true as I navigated my grief: "Only people who are capable of loving strongly can also suffer great sorrow, but this same necessity of loving serves to counteract their grief and heals them." Fyodor Dostoyevsky suggested something similar: "The darker the night, the brighter the stars, the deeper the grief, the closer is God!"

The "good grief" cycle

"Good grief" sounds like an oxymoron—two contrasting ideas that don't quite fit together. In reality, however, there is such a thing as good grief. It is good grief that heals those who are wounded and sorrowing because of life's losses. Good grief includes positive elements that keep us from getting stuck or stalled indefinitely when we grieve. Good grief involves leaning into the pain of loss and learning more about ourselves and others as a result.

Our understanding of the grief cycle grew out of the work certain doctors did after suffering embarrassment when their terminally ill patients died. When the patients died, the doctors treating them felt like failures. They started shunning the dying because they didn't think there was anything else they could do to help them. One doctor, however, felt differently. Elisabeth Kübler-

Ross, a doctor in Switzerland, challenged this unkindness and spent time with dying people, both comforting and studying them. Then she wrote a book called *On Death and Dying*, which included a description of the emotional states grieving people go through, sometimes referred to as the grief cycle. As time went on, it was noticed that this emotional cycle was not just experienced by the dying, but also by people affected by any kind of negative change or loss, such as losing a job. The grief cycle includes five emotional states:

- **Denial or shock** — avoidance, confusion, fear, blame
- **Anger** — frustration, anxiety, irritation, shame
- **Depression** — detachment, blahs, lack of energy, helplessness
- **Bargaining** — dialogue, reaching out to others, a desire to tell your story
- **Acceptance** — exploring options, a new plan

Grief observed firsthand

Our accident and the recovery process that followed created an opportunity for "good grief." All of us touched by this traumatic event needed to grieve, including our family and friends. The range of emotions associated with the loss was broad and ever changing. The grief was anything but neat and tidy.

When I woke up two days after the accident, I was in shock and disbelief at what had happened. I was in a fog and numb to the full impact of the loss and damage that had occurred. I remember the frustration I felt — and the shame. I blamed myself for what had happened. After all, I had been driving the motorcycle. "If only..." ran through my head several times. There were waves of depression that came and went, depending on the news I received in any given week. I lacked energy and felt helpless at times. I lacked motivation when called upon to fight and claw my way back to health. I reached out to others continuously and found ways to tell my story to anyone who would listen. At the five-month mark,

I had a memorable breakthrough in accepting my loss. It was not the last time I'd need to accept what I had lost, but it was one milestone I marked while on my detour. The acceptance came as a willingness to go the distance with my recovery, no matter how long it took.

To be honest, my grief was messier than it sounds and came and went in waves. In the early stages, I experienced grief "lite" while after a few more surgeries, months of immobility, and long periods when I was unable to work, I experienced grief "advanced."

Practices that kept me moving in my grief

For me, the key to having "good" grief was to keep moving. There were a few practical ways I kept my grief going when part of me wanted to give up.

One practice was to be brutally honest with myself instead of trying to be tough and unaffected by the pain and loss. A Turkish proverb says, "He who conceals his grief finds no remedy for it."

Another practice was to share my pain with trustworthy friends. A French proverb puts it this way: "Friendship doubles our joy and divides our grief." I tried to be open to reflecting on and learning from my own pain and the pain of others. Benjamin Franklin wrote, "Those things that hurt, instruct."

I prayed the book of Psalms. The Psalms put into words what I couldn't articulate and helped me process my pain and suffering. I personalized the prayers in the Psalms and made them my prayers: "I went through fire and water, but you brought me to a place of abundance."[32]

Another practice was to be patient and not try to rush the time I needed to grieve. Shakespeare said, "Grief makes one hour ten." The days were sometimes long and the nights longer, but I learned to slow down and travel at a new speed.

Other practices were to have a greater purpose and to shed tears. Viktor E. Frankl mentored me on both points. He wrote, "Life is never made unbearable by circumstances, but only by lack of meaning and purpose" and "But there was no need to be ashamed of tears, for tears bore witness that a man had the greatest of courage, the courage to suffer."

The four tasks of grief

John Adams observed, "Grief drives men into habits of serious reflection, sharpens the understanding, and softens the heart." A framework I found life giving as I worked through my grief was "the tasks of grief" developed by William Worden:[33]

1. Accept the reality of the loss.

This task is to come to terms with the fact that life as you knew it is over. When a loved one dies, when an opportunity is lost, when an activity can no longer be enjoyed, or when a dream is broken, acceptance is essential to moving forward.

I had to accept the loss of work opportunities, let go of my love of running, and give up the freedom to come and go as I pleased (for a long while). Those losses loomed large in the beginning, but as I accepted my situation one piece at a time, I found myself inching along in my healing.

2. Experience the pain of grief.

Grieving is an emotional roller coaster. The key is to experience the pain of grief, not just think about it. You must go down into the emotional quagmire of anger, loneliness, depression, frustration, disappointment, and sadness.

If I had avoided the emotions of loss or minimized what I was experiencing, I would have delayed the pain but seen the same emotions resurface in unhealthy ways later on. C.S. Lewis, reflecting on his grief, said, "No one ever told me that grief felt so like fear."

3. Adjust to the new environment.

This third task is to get used to the new reality without whatever or whomever you've lost. You may have more responsibility, less mobility, fewer options, or a change in status. Adjusting practically to what you now have to work with is what this stage is all about.

I had to adjust to being alone at home in my recliner from Monday to Friday. I had to adjust to a serious downgrade in the options available to me for how to occupy my time. My world had suddenly shrunk in size, and I had to adjust my expectations to meet my new reality. That was true early on and also as recovery progressed in the later stages.

4. Reinvest energy in life.

The fourth task is to lean into new activities and relationships that fit with your new reality. This includes learning to love and relate to new people, finding purpose in your adjusted activities, and valuing the new things that you have discovered have meaning for you.

I gave myself permission to laugh and live again. I shed tears of joy when I thought about the quality friendships I had and how I had encouraged people I hadn't even met. I learned to get outside every day on my scooter, breathe in the fresh air, listen to the creek trickle by, and look for new ways to live. A Chinese proverb concludes, "One joy shatters a hundred griefs."

Tears and the healing process

According to Ecclesiastes 3:4, there is "a time to laugh," but there is also "a time to cry." A Jewish saying advises, "What soap is for the body, tears are for the soul." Tears were soap for my soul many times.

Not all tears are created equal. According to researchers, "Crying is often beneficial, but benefits may depend on the traits of the crier, their social support system, and whether the crier has ongoing psychological problems like depression or anxiety."[34] In other words, those with anxiety and those unable to experience pleasure are the least likely to benefit from crying.

Some people see tears as a sign of weakness, and because of that the healing process is hindered in them. Some people fear what will be unleashed if they ever start to cry, and that fear holds them back from the deeper healing that tears can bring. But tears can be a good friend and a sign of strength. In my recovery, tears helped me heal in several ways:

- **Tears helped me cope with the pain of loss.**

Shakespeare said, "To weep is to make less the depth of grief." Had I run from the pain of loss, I would have missed the healing power that tears brought.

- **Tears kept me healthy.**

Crying removed toxins from my body.

- **Tears lowered my stress levels.**

Tears aren't just salt water. They contain an endorphin that modulates pain, as well as hormones that have been released during times of stress. William Frey explains that crying "flushes excess and toxic stress hormones" from the body.

- **Tears connected me to God.**

When I prayed the Psalms, I found myself connecting deeply with God, who I sensed understood and accepted my raw emotion. I identified with David, who said to God, "You've kept track of my every toss and turn through the sleepless nights, each tear entered in your ledger, each ache written in your book."[35]

Grief counselor Dr. Lou LaGrand said, "Tears communicate, lubricate, elicit sympathy, change mood, reduce tension, and help us cope with a multitude of losses throughout life. The therapeutic value of crying is clear: accept, encourage, and nurture crying in yourself as well as those you support in times of change. Don't rush for the Kleenex. Let a good cry happen."[36]

A lesson from two rivers

When you drive through Lytton, BC, you can see the muddy Fraser River meeting the clean Thompson River. This is called a "confluence," which means "flowing together." To me, that is a metaphor for the journey of grief. When we are grieving, two contrasting parts of life touch each other — the muddy, difficult part and the clean, bright parts. One moment we're up to our neck in sadness, loss, disappointment, pain, and frustration. The next moment we're witnessing a brilliant sunset, enjoying the company of close friends, or making a memory with our kids.

The challenge during times of grief is to keep the muddy losses from overtaking everything clean and bright in our life. The muddy Fraser River does eventually overtake the clean Thompson, but it doesn't need to be that way in life. We do not need to be in a perpetual state of sadness and frustration. Instead, we can learn to hold onto both streams at the same time.

People would call on me and ask me how I was doing. If it was a muddy day or week, I'd tell them but also include what I was thankful for or what I was hoping for. When I asked them how they were doing, if they were about to travel to an amazing place, they would often feel guilty for the pleasurable experience they were about to have.

The guilt we feel when we pull back from embracing positive emotion is false guilt, stemming from the awkwardness of trying to hold muddy water and clear water simultaneously. The goal is to fully embrace, separately, the moments of fun and pleasure and the moments of loss, sadness, and pain.

Detour Reflections

❖ What in your experience has helped you experience "good grief"?

❖ What has kept you stuck in the process of grief?

Chapter 13: Forgiveness

Forgiveness is "me giving up my right to hurt you for hurting me." If you want to live free and avoid the pain and suffering that result from unforgiveness, give up your right to hurt the people who have hurt you. Glenn Clark advised, "If you wish to travel far and fast, travel light. Take off all your envies, jealousies, unforgiveness, selfishness, and fears."

It was two years before Vicky and I traveled back to the scene of our accident, just thirty minutes from our home. We waited two years, not because we couldn't face it but because we just weren't mobile enough to travel. The visit to the scene was one we knew we needed to make even with the mixture of emotions it would inevitably create.

Going back to the corner of Johnson Road and Highway 7 reminded me of my brokenness and the hurt caused by driver error. One man's inattentiveness changed our lives and the trajectory of where we were headed. We lost a lot that day, but I came to realize soon afterwards that if I wanted to heal, I needed to give up my right to hurt the person who hurt me. It wasn't easy, but I knew I had to forgive.

The benefits of forgiveness

The benefits of forgiveness are many, regardless of the source of the hurt. When we forgive, it has a positive impact on our own lives. What are the benefits of choosing to forgive? Below are a few that I have noticed.

1.   When we forgive, we heal broken relationships.

The biblical story of Joseph is a powerful story of forgiveness. Joseph's brothers hated him and sold him into slavery. Years later, Joseph had risen to one of the highest positions in the Egyptian government. He was reintroduced to his brothers when they came to Egypt looking for food in the midst of a famine. Joseph recognized his brothers, but they had no idea he was still alive. Instead of wanting to hurt them for what they had done to him, he forgave them, wept in their presence, and saw healing in his family. Joseph said these powerful words: "Don't be afraid of me. Am I God, that I can punish you? You intended to harm me, but God intended it all for good. He brought me to this position so I could save the lives of many people."[37]

2. When we forgive, we grow in character.

Character is forged in the fire of adversity. Forgiving someone who has hurt us can be extremely difficult, but when we exercise forgiveness, we end up growing on the inside. Proverbs 19:11 (NIV) says, "A person's wisdom yields patience; it is to one's glory to overlook an offense."

There are situations where forgiveness seems impossible. The hurt is so deep and so devastating that we just can't seem to let it go. At those moments, we need inner strength of character. Mahatma Gandhi said, "The weak can never forgive. Forgiveness is the attribute of the strong."

3. When we forgive, we experience physical and emotional health.

Studies show that forgiveness results in a better immune system, lower blood pressure, better mental health, lower amounts of anger, and fewer symptoms of anxiety and depression. When I think about the challenges I had fighting infection and climbing back out of the deep pit I was in, I realize how much harder it would have been if I had been carrying a load of bitterness and resentment.

Unforgiveness imprisons us in resentment and bitterness and erodes the soul. The process of forgiving might take a while, but it is a trip worth taking. Suzanne Somers said, "Forgiveness is a gift you give yourself."

Forgiveness is a decision to ACT a certain way

Forgiveness starts in the heart and works its way out to the fringes of our lives. It is a journey that has varying degrees of messiness and difficultly depending on the nature of the hurt. The accident had hurt me on multiple levels—emotionally, physically, psychologically, spiritually, and vocationally. The good news for me was that I forgave the person who caused our hurt. I prayed for his well-being and did not wish any harm to come upon him. I made the following decisions to ACT in ways that helped me walk through the journey of forgiveness.

1. Admit you have been hurt.

Denial is the pathway to bitterness and loneliness. Owning up to your pain and hurt sets you on the road towards healing. When you admit your hurt, healing starts, which leads to the ability to help others.

One of the ways to know that people are admitting they are hurt is that they are willing to talk about their pain. Healing will not happen if you don't get through this stage of admitting your hurt. If you stay in denial, the cycle of hurt will continue because "hurt people hurt people."

2. Choose to forgive.

Once you have admitted you were hurt, you can take the next step. That step is to acknowledge the need to forgive and then follow through. That is, you must agree to pay the price in time, vulnerability, and effort in order to release the need to hurt the person who hurt you. Choosing to forgive begins in your head, moves into your heart, and is then carried out in your actions.

My journey of choosing to forgive the person who hurt me started with calling out to God for help. He met me in my weakness and gave me the strength and courage to forgive. I also had people I could talk with to help me work through the process.

3. Take the time and trouble to be fully healed.

Sometimes the process of forgiveness includes speaking to the person who hurt you. I never did speak to the person who had hurt me, but I would have if I had felt it was necessary. I arrived at that decision after some soul searching and heeded the wisdom of my therapist, who didn't feel it was essential.

Becoming fully healed takes time and effort. In some situations, forgiving too quickly short-circuits the healing process and robs you of the peace you need to move on. You know you're healed when you no longer hold a grudge, when your attitude, your behavior, your emotional condition, and the way you speak about the other person reflects the heart of a person who has let it go.

Harry's story

On February 24, 1948, one of the most unusual operations in medical history took place at Ohio State University. A stony sheath was removed from around the heart of thirty-year-old Harry Besharra. As a boy, he had been shot accidentally by a friend with a .22 rifle, and the bullet had remained lodged in his heart. The bullet had not killed him, but a lime deposit had started to slowly form over his heart, strangling this vital organ. In the surgery, the doctor separated Harry's ribs, moved the left lung to the side, and peeled off the stony coating around the heart, like peeling an orange. Immediately, the pressure on the heart was reduced, and it started to pump normally. When Harry awoke from surgery, he was asked how he felt. His response was, "I feel 1,000 percent better already!"

The lesson in Harry's story is this: When we experience hurt, over time our hearts can form a hard, protective coating. When that happens, life starts to get choked out of us, and surgery is required.

My story

There was one day during my recovery when I knew I needed to get out of the house and go for a short walk. At that point in my recovery, just walking to the end of the street and back was an achievement. On this particular day, I could feel my heart tighten up and my mind struggle with the awkwardness and challenge of each step. I sensed a stirring of resentment and disappointment in my soul. I found myself longing for the good old days when I could walk and run without giving it a second thought. I knew those days were long gone, but I still heard myself whispering, "Why did this have to happen?" The thought didn't last long or go very deep because I knew in that moment I had to make a choice to let the past go and to be thankful for what I had and the progress I was making. I knew I couldn't let a stony coating of resentment, bitterness, and hard-heartedness form and squeeze the life out of me.

If we allow the stony deposit of unforgiveness to settle into our hearts and minds, it will choke out our joy, diminish our passion, and steal away our life. I learned to remain open to repeated minor heart surgeries to keep any crusty residue from forming. Stephen Covey observed, "The greatest battles of life are fought out every day in the silent chambers of our own heart."

Final thought

There is no cookie cutter approach to forgiveness and keeping your heart clear from calluses. I remember the 832nd day after the accident when I discovered some residue on my heart that needed to be removed. I was shocked, but realized again that the journey of forgiveness is never over but continues throughout our lives.

Detour Reflections

❖ What do you do to process the hurt and pain caused by the injuries of others?

❖ Is there anyone you need to give up the right to hurt because of the hurt they caused you? What is the next step you need to take to fully forgive?

Chapter 14: Perseverance

How you start matters, but how you finish matters even more. In order to finish well, perseverance is required. Perseverance is "steady persistence in a course of action, a purpose, a state, etc., especially in spite of difficulties, obstacles, or discouragement."[38]

Perseverance is an inner quality developed one choice at a time. Julia Cameron said, "Often it is tenacity, not talent, that rules the day." Titus Lucretius Carus underlined the power of perseverance when he said, "Constant dripping hollows out a stone." Albert Einstein put it another way when he said that genius is "1 percent talent and 99 percent hard work."

Days I needed perseverance the most

Perseverance was as necessary as oxygen during my detour. It was the muscle I used regularly to overcome difficulties, obstacles, and discouragement and to keep going when the minutes turned into hours, the hours turned into days, the days turned into months, and the months turned into years.

There were many days when I called upon perseverance. Six of those days stand out.

Day 139

On Labor Day, 2011, I checked myself back into Royal Columbian Hospital (RCH). I was following the advice of an emergency room doctor at Abbotsford Hospital who had told me, "You need to go back to RCH and have them look at this problem since they know your case." At RCH, the medical staff took a look, tested my blood, and instantly concluded I was in trouble and in need of more surgery. There was an abscess in my leg, caused by the same infection I had had originally.

When I had left RCH on day 21, I (along with the doctors) had believed that the six weeks of antibiotics I was on would be enough to deal with the infection. As spring had turned into summer, I had continued with what I thought was a normal recovery—yet all was not well. All summer I had struggled with pain. I would wake up in the night wet with sweat. I was thin and gaunt, I found physiotherapy an uphill battle, and I was always tired.

The truth came out when I returned to RCH on day 136. That week, I was assigned to an infectious disease doctor who would figure out what bacteria I was dealing with and what antibiotic would be required to fight it. She discovered that the bacteria I had was normally found in manure pits but rarely found in humans and was challenging to kill.

On day 139, I had my first surgery with lower body reconstruction specialist Dr. Viskontas. I didn't know it at the time, but he was exactly the help I needed for the long road ahead.

Day 201

On day 201, Dr. Viskontas removed six inches of my right femur. It had to come out because the infection had moved into the bone. It was a choice between removing the leg and cutting out the bone. Thankfully, my surgeon chose the latter.

To hold the femur in place, an external fixator was attached with pins to the two remaining sections of the femur, and a cement spacer was inserted into the gap where the bone had come out. After the surgery, I went back on antibiotics for another six weeks, and I prayed that this round would kill the bacteria once and for all. I didn't want to lose my leg, but all I could do was hope and persevere.

While I was recovering from this surgery, I was inspired to persevere by the story of fourteen-year-old Bethany Hamilton, who had her arm bitten off by a shark. She wrote: "What I do know is that I want to use what happened to me as an opportunity to tell people that God is worthy of our trust, and to show them that you can go on and do wonderful things in spite of terrible events that happen."

I called day 205 my "horrific day." I was still recovering from surgery in RCH when my leg filled up with fluid, which pushed me to a "10" on the pain scale. The doctor came in to see what was happening. He opted to give me morphine and more oxycodone and let me ride it out instead of draining the fluid and running the risk of further infection. I persevered and somehow made it through that hiccup.

Day 286

Day 286 was scheduled to be the day to take off the external fixator so I could begin the process of regrowing the femur. Unfortunately, that plan had to wait. When Dr. Viskontas opened up the leg, he found dead tissue, an indication that the infection might still be a threat.

This surgery had an interesting twist—I was awake for much of it. The reason for that was that the anesthetic they used was a spinal, which didn't put me to sleep as a general anesthetic would have. While I lay there on the hard metal table listening to what was going on, I was given a perfect opportunity for my perseverance muscle to grow stronger. I heard the chatter of the surgical team and the noise of the drill removing the fixator. I heard the sound of the mallet pounding a cement-coated nail down through my hip and into my femur. Then I heard "Oh, shit!" (It is never a good sign to hear a comment like that when you are in the middle of surgery.)

The days that followed brought pain, weariness, light-headedness (due to a low hemoglobin count), tears, endless waiting—but also tons of support. I wondered when my ordeal would end, but all I could do was press on. When a friend asked me how I was doing, I replied, "I feel like a piece of sheet metal torn off a roof in a windstorm."

Day 375

Finally, the day came when the infection was gone and the next step in the rebuilding process could be taken. In my case, it was time to regrow my femur with a bone transporter. Bone transporters come in various shapes and sizes. They are used to "stretch legs" or grow legs longer in children born with one leg shorter than the other.

On day 375, Dr. Viskontas opened up my leg and installed the bone transporter. I was a novelty around the hospital as it is rare for an adult to have a bone transporter. Even some of the nurses had never seen what I was wearing.

The bone transporter was a piece of black metal about fourteen inches long that was attached to the outside of my right femur. Two pins were screwed through my leg into the part of the femur that came down from my hip, and two pins were attached to the part of the femur that came up from my knee. In between was a five-inch gap that eventually would be filled with new bone. Down the middle of the femur, was a metal rod that extended the complete length of the femur.

The new bone growth took place inside my leg between two pieces of healthy bone. Broken bones heal by growing new bone marrow to fill in the space created. That same natural process was used to grow a new section of my femur. The crack was created by breaking off a three inch section of healthy femur and sliding it down the rod with the help of two pins attached to the outside bracket. I used an Allen key to turn a screw four quarter-turns per day, equaling one millimeter. That movement kept the piece of bone far enough ahead of the gap to stimulate new bone growth.

It was a fascinating but awful experience.

The growth of the bone produced the worst pain of the entire detour. The two pins cut a path through the leg as they moved the unattached piece of bone down the internal rod. In addition, the piece of bone was pushing against muscle fibre, blood vessels, and other soft tissue as it moved down the inside of the leg.

It took perseverance and tenacity to complete the process.

Day 549

What a relief it was to get the bone transporter off! The hardware had done its work, and it was time to say goodbye to it. Of course, I wasn't done quite yet. I had to wait for the new bone to calcify and grow strong enough before I could begin putting my weight on that leg.

As I waited and continued to press forward on the detour, I filled my mind and soul with positive words and thoughts. One day, I received a text that included an old Irish proverb: "Hope is the physician of each misery." The text also said:

Oh, may our longing to kneel always be greater than our longing to be healed…never choose despair when you can choose hope. Despair will never bolster you, support you, or encourage you. It will begin your slow demise…Hope says, "He who limps is still walking." Hope will ground you, anchor you, and make you unshakable.

I couldn't put much weight on my right leg for several weeks as I waited for the new bone to harden from one end to the other. I lived with a knee that had atrophied because of lying dormant for so long. I still couldn't drive, but I spent my days staying busy, with very little mobility but with an increasing capacity to be engaged in mind and heart.

I enjoyed scooter rides by the stream, writing projects I could work on in my recliner, visits with friends who stopped by, lunch with my father-in-law on my way home from having more X-rays taken, sports on TV, books that could be read, podcasts that could be listened to, and journaling that needed to be completed.

Day 1004

The last major surgery seemed to take forever to arrive. This, my ninth surgery, gave me greater range of motion in my knee—from 80 degrees to around 120 degrees (eventually).

Day 1004 found me in a taxi early in the morning, so I could be at RCH in time for surgery. I felt like an experienced surgical patient as I was wheeled into the operating room. I knew what to expect and what had been planned for the surgery. I was prepared for three procedures—a knee release, a quadricepsplasty (a procedure to pull the quadriceps muscle away from the femur so the knee could bend farther), and a tibial tubercle osteotomy (a repositioning of the patella or knee cap). Dr. Viskontas arranged to have a knee specialist partner with him during the surgery to increase the chances of success.

The surgery started with five failed attempts to administer an epidural, which itself produced serious discomfort. The anesthesiologist ended up giving me a general anesthetic, which put me right out.

When the surgery was over, I woke up as usual in the recovery room next to the operating room. I took some comfort in hearing that the surgery had gone well and that the tibial tubercle osteotomy had not been needed. I was shocked, however, to be greeted by a physiotherapist in the recovery room—while I was still pushing the morphine pump and sipping on ice cubes to quench my thirst. At the sight of the physiotherapist, my inside voice said, "There is no rest for the recovering soul. What's a physiotherapist doing here?" The physiotherapist was there to strap a continuous passive motion (CPM) machine onto my right leg. It was an ingenious device that kept my knee bending back and forth, automatically, twenty-four hours a day, seven days a week. Without it, the quadriceps muscle that had just been unstuck from my femur would reattach and nullify the surgery's impact.

I persevered. When I went home a few days later, I was fitted with a home version of the CPM, and for thirty days I stayed tied to that machine twenty-three hours per day. I would carry the CPM to bed with me at night so my knee would keep moving.

I eventually said goodbye to the CPM and persevered to do the work necessary to grow stronger every day. I never quit believing I would get through this, and even though I didn't know what my new normal would look like, I pressed on, continuing to strengthen my perseverance muscle.

Six strategies for working the perseverance muscle

Enduring when the days were long and the nights were longer required both a positive attitude and a plan. More effort didn't always help. Sometimes I needed a new direction, a new perspective, or a new strategy. Perseverance is an attitude that needs a strategy to go with it. Perseverance believes things will get better eventually but learns to deal with the brutal facts and realities faced on a regular basis.

1. Be fully present where you are.

I didn't always want to be where I was, but I realized if I fought against where I was, I would remain stuck much longer. Henry Cloud said: "Living in the present will make your stress go down and your happiness go up. Even if the present is sad, to embrace those feelings is part of having them pass. Feelings we avoid, get stuck in our system and will return until we face them, so whether in good times or bad, the lesson is to be 'in time.' Be there, in the now."[39]

2. Be grateful even on the darkest days.

Gratitude expressed changes the way we feel and the way we see the world. When I intentionally looked for and found ways to be grateful, I found myself inching forward just a little.

Henry Ward Beecher said, "The unthankful heart discovers no mercies; but the thankful heart will find, in every hour, some heavenly blessings." I never stopped thanking God for the people he brought into my life to help me. I was practicing the advice John F. Kennedy gave: "We must find time to stop and thank the people who make a difference in our lives."

3. Be a curious learner.

Curiosity and learning go together. I never stopped learning and being curious about what was going on all around me or what needed to change within me. Even when my mind was in a fog or I was completely exhausted, I learned what I could and passed it on. When interns looked at my bone transporter and my X-rays in the cast clinic, they would often have questions. I always enjoyed answering some of their questions, based on what I had learned by observations, asking good questions, and research.

4. Breathe deeply.

Perseverance is a journey, not a destination. On the detour, I learned to stop to smell the flowers, smile as the dogs chased the birds, and take deep breaths as I rode my scooter by the path alongside the stream. On some days, I stayed too long in the house and knew I needed to get outside and breathe some fresh air. When I did, it changed my view and my mood. There is a Swedish proverb that says, "Fear less, hope more. Eat less, chew more. Whine less, breathe more."

5. Take baby steps.

How did I get from day 136 to day 1004? Baby steps. I learned to tackle one surgery at a time, one physio session at a time, one bag of antibiotics at a time, one needle at a time, one painkiller at a time. Perseverance is best served in bite-sized pieces. Be near-sighted. Take one day at a time. Take one hour at a time. Take one minute at a time. Take one baby step at a time.

6. Process your emotions.

When we are in pain or going through a rough patch, emotions will bubble up from the inside—including anger, frustration, sadness, disappointment, and fear. One strategy I used to process my emotions was journaling. It helped me flush out and flesh out what was going on inside. I also processed emotions by talking to trusted friends, talking to God, and letting the tears flow.

Final thought

Brad Gast wrote, "No matter what happens, no matter how far you seem to be away from where you want to be, never stop believing that you will somehow make it. Have an unrelenting belief that things will work out, that the long road has a purpose, that the things that you desire may not happen today, but they will happen. Continue to persist and persevere."[40]

Detour Reflections

❖ Where do you need perseverance the most in your life?

❖ What habit do you need to develop in order to strengthen your perseverance muscle?

Chapter 15: Attitude

Like the attitude indicator on the dashboard of an airplane, our attitude reveals the orientation of our life compared to our surroundings. If our attitude is pointing in a downward direction, a crash is coming. If our attitude is pointed in a skyward direction, we will soar. Our attitude is not dependent on the weather but rather is a perspective we choose regardless of the weather. It is true that people can be predisposed to a positive or negative attitude because of personality or conditioning. The good news is that we can change our attitude.

Over the years, I intentionally cultivated an optimistic attitude, and during my recovery it served me well. An upward pointing attitude is not based on brains, wealth, luck, beauty, athleticism, or circumstances. It is based on believing good can come out of bad, present pain can eventually lead to future healing, and there is a way to redeem something of value out of challenging circumstances. My attitude mentor Zig Ziglar once said, "Your attitude, not your aptitude, will determine your altitude."

An attitude adjustment story

Following surgery number five, I visited the cast clinic so my surgeon and those assisting him could remove the staples and sutures and see how I was doing. To my surprise, the doctor exclaimed, "Oh, God!" when he saw my leg. Coming from him, this was a little shocking as he wasn't known for showing emotion or being shocked by anything. Dr. Viskontas had looked over my X-rays, observed how the healing was going, and noticed how much shorter my right leg actually was compared to earlier estimates. What had been a five-millimeter difference in leg length was now estimated to be twenty-five millimeters; that is, my right leg was a

DETOUR

full inch shorter than the left leg. I was shocked. I felt my attitude take a nosedive as the reality sank in.

Shortly after that, a shift in my attitude started to happen. I began to reflect on the fact that I still had a leg and the fact that there were shoe lifts that could correct the problem. As I shifted my attitude, the bad news no longer seemed as devastating as it had at first, and I was able to start moving forward again. An upwardly pointing attitude had given me the lift I needed to step back and see the bigger picture. Did it happen instantaneously? Not at all. It was a gradual adjustment.

Part of what had prepared me to adjust my attitude was the grieving I had done a week earlier immediately following that particular surgery. A soaring attitude said, "I have a leg and a future even if it comes with a limp." A soaring attitude paved the way for inner peace that helped me to rise above my circumstances. A soaring attitude fueled my ability to press on in spite of my limitations. I was looking at what was left, not at what I had lost. The result was more energy to focus on getting better. This same attitude helped me come to terms later on with the fact that my right leg was actually sixty-five millimeters (two and a half inches) shorter than my left leg.

Five actions that fan the flame of positivity

You cultivate a soaring attitude when you practice positivity — even when there are those in your life who are negative and try to throw a wet blanket over your positivity. You cannot control what others do around you, but you can control how you respond to your circumstances. There are at least five actions I used to counter negativity.

1. Make your room great.

You may not be able to control the temperature in the whole house around you, but you can control the temperature in your own room — the place where you play, your specific role at work, the place where you serve, your circle of friends, and the inputs you allow to enter your life through your eyes and ears. Every day, when I woke up, my goal was to do something positive with the time I had and to find a way to add value to others. I had the freedom to sit in front of the TV all day, eat barbecue chips, and let life pass me by. But that would not have contributed to making my room great. I learned to tune out the negativity around me and stay focused on what I could control.

2. Differentiate melancholy from negativity.

A lot of "positive talk" fails to acknowledge the presence of legitimate loss and the emotional roller coaster that inevitably comes with adversity. If your positivity is a fluffy sentimentalism that says, "Let's just be happy all the time," it's not the positivity I'm talking about. My positivity had room for melancholy and sadness as an unavoidable part of human experience.

The positivity I'm talking about is not the absence of adversity but a belief that you'll get through what you're going through, that people will show up to help at just the right time, and that there are resources you haven't yet tapped into (including divine aid). Real positivity believes in growth amidst hardship and fights against the downward pull of the feeling that life will never get better and nobody cares.

3. Be the change you want to see.

Mahatma Gandhi famously said, "Be the change you want to see in the world." The change I wanted to see was that I would be positive and hopeful in all my speaking, thinking, praying, believing, and responding. I learned to avoid being pulled down by the negativity surrounding me. I chose to focus on positive self-talk, the good, the best, the pure, and the beautiful. Negativity is a powerful force, but I learned that I could also be powerful when I let my light shine brightly. I learned to live with true hope that said, "Things can and will get better!"

4. Invite others to join you.

You can't directly change other people, but you can change yourself—and, by doing that, you just might influence others to choose to make their own change. If your life radiates a peaceful spirit, a strong faith, a persevering attitude, and kind words and actions, others will take notice. There is something magnetic about people who live what they believe and boldly invite others to join them in that way of living. Positive people make an upward-pointing attitude believable.

5. If others fail to join you, press on.

Positivity believes in a bright future and the difference one life can make. No one is born with a positive attitude. Some people are more optimistic by temperament, but, no matter who you are, you can cultivate positivity by practicing it every single day.

Throughout the toughest days of my detour, I learned to focus on what brought life instead of on what drained me of energy and optimism. When surgeries revealed more problems, when my recovery was met by major setbacks, when work opportunities vanished into thin air, I focused on what I had left and who I wanted to be that day.

Attitudes you can't live without

There were certain attitudes I adopted that gave me courage and inner fortitude to keep going. I didn't always maintain the attitudes I describe here, but they gave me ideals to strive for and helped me stay on track most of the time.

1. The long view is worth the trip.

If I had fixated on the short term, I would have missed seeing the deeper work that was going on within me. Shortsightedness during times of adversity leads to missed lessons and missed discoveries. Haruki Murakami wrote,

Once the storm is over, you won't remember how you made it through, how you managed to survive. You won't even be sure whether the storm is really over. But one thing is certain. When you come out of the storm, you won't be the same person who walked in. That's what this storm's all about.[41]

2. Pain nourishes courage.

Courage is both an attitude and a muscle that grows stronger when exercised. When you act courageous, you become courageous. When I faced my pain and suffering head on, I grew my courage to keep going. Mary Tyler Moore said, "Pain nourishes courage. You can't be brave if you've only had wonderful things happen to you."

3. Normalizing adversity lowers stress and creates opportunity.

Unrealistic expectations increase stress. When I accepted difficulty as part of my life on this planet, my stress decreased, and I actually created space in my heart and mind to see new possibilities. Paralympian Aimee Mullins said, "There's a partnership between perceived deficiencies and our creative ability, so it's not about sweeping under the rug the challenges but finding the opportunity wrapped in the adversity…Perhaps if we see adversity as natural, consistent and useful, we're less burdened by the presence of it."[42]

4. Commitment strengthens the resolve to keep going.

When I made a conscious decision to not give up but to press on regardless of what came, my resolve grew stronger. Joel Osteen taught, "You must make a decision that you are going to move on. It won't happen automatically. You will have to rise up and say, 'I don't care how hard this is, I don't care how disappointed I am. I'm not going to let this get the best of me. I'm moving on with my life.'"

5. Inner beauty is formed through trials.

If I entered my right leg in a beauty contest, I'd lose. It's scarred, sunken, and short, but that's only half the story. Real beauty is who we are on the inside, in our character. My scars tell a story of inner change and growth in character. Elisabeth Kübler-Ross wrote, "The most beautiful people I've known are those who have known trials, have known struggles, have known loss, and have found their way out of the depths."

6. Difficulty turns up the volume on our ability to hear God speak.

I believe it's worth the time and trouble to pay attention to anything God says. He knows me best and has incredible wisdom I don't want to miss, especially during the hard times. As C.S. Lewis once said, "God whispers to us in our pleasure, speaks to us in our conscience, but shouts to us in our pain."

7. Hardship creates a powerful learning laboratory.

A long time ago, I decided to be a lifelong learner. Having that settled in my mind allowed me to be all ears and eyes during my detour so I could pick up the lessons I needed to learn. Mark Twain said, "A person who has had a bull by the tail once has learned sixty to seventy times as much as a person who hasn't."

8. Calamity tears away nonessentials and leaves what really matters.

During the detour, I looked back on my life and noticed I had spent a lot of time chasing nonessentials. The suffering during the detour uncovered what really mattered and exposed the nonessentials for what they really were. Arthur Golden said, "Adversity is like a strong wind. It tears away from us all but the things that cannot be torn, so that we see ourselves as we really are."

9. Hard times show true character.

My character has always been under construction. However, during the pressure of hard times, the true colors of my character came out into the light. A valuable takeaway during the detour was that I should always be ready for my character to show up well under pressure. James 1:3 (MSG) says, "You know that under pressure, your faith-life is forced into the open and shows its true colors."

10. Adversity is a pathway to success.

Two words I started pairing together during my detour were "success" and "adversity." True success is impossible without adversity. Zig Ziglar said, "Sometimes adversity is what you need to face in order to become successful."

Detour Reflections

❖ How do you describe your predisposition to life?

❖ What can you do on a daily basis to fan the flame of positivity in your life?

Chapter 16: Expectations

Expectations can be our friend or our enemy. They are our friend when the final outcome matches what we had hoped for. They are our enemy when the outcome is nowhere close to what we had imagined it would be.

On my roller roaster ride of expectations, I tried, with some success, to stay out of two ditches. One ditch had no expectations. The other ditch had completely unrealistic expectations. The first ditch sounds simple but is mythical in nature and does not provide enough push to promote healthy growth. Alexander Pope could not have been farther from the truth when he said, "Blessed is he who expects nothing, for he shall never be disappointed." The second ditch leaves us equally empty because when our plans don't match our capacity to achieve, we are left reeling in unbelief. This second ditch was where I found myself one day in the physiotherapy clinic.

The day my expectations got smashed

Physiotherapy had been progressing nicely for some time. As I stood in the hall of the physiotherapy clinic this particular day, it was time for some show and tell. My physiotherapist began to explain my situation to a colleague, which included taking a good look at the scar on my right leg. The scar is quite a nasty sight as a result of multiple surgeries and the reconstruction that was required to deal with the infection. Much of the quad muscle was not even working at that point.

The good news was that I was making process. I was able to put about 75 percent of my weight on my right leg, my ankle was rotating well, and the quad muscle was getting stronger with each rep. The bad news was that I could only bend my knee about 85 degrees. To put that in perspective, to turn a bike pedal normally, I would need at least 110 degrees of bend. That meant that I would have to come to terms with the fact that I would need another round of painful knee bending by the physiotherapist to extend the range of motion. It was also clear that another painful surgery was in my future, in order to increase the range of motion to 120 degrees.

I didn't deal with my reality very well at all that day — and my struggle was directly tied to my expectations. I was not where I thought I should be. Because my expectations had not been met, I was overwhelmed with melancholy, tears, and frustration.

What had I expected to be doing by then? I had expected to be driving. I had expected to be bending my knee more than 100 degrees. I had expected the leg to be able to bear my full weight. I had expected to be able to avoid another knee surgery *somehow*. I had expected to be more energized and not to be so tired from all this rehab! I had expected this whole ordeal to be a lot easier than it actually was.

The recipe I followed to adjust my expectations to my reality

There were a few key ingredients I mixed together to produce a set of more realistic expectations. This realignment helped get me back on track. Finding realistic expectations made the difference between misery and peace.

Ingredient #1: A cup of honesty

The search for realistic expectations starts with honest self-reflection. I had to look in the mirror and be honest about what I saw and felt. I had to admit my sadness and disappointment and tell those closest to me that I had been wrong about where I was at. I talked to my wife, close friends, and others who could help me speak the difficult truth out loud and look squarely at reality .

Admitting we are in a dark tunnel is a bit like admitting we have a toothache. We won't get help until we admit we have a problem. Honesty is the foundation on which we can build more realistic expectations. Honesty includes being honest with God, who is more than able to handle any amount of frustration and disappointment.

Ingredient #2: A pound of control

After honesty came the realization that if I focused on what I could control, I could start to climb out of the funk in which I found myself. I asked myself, "What can I do to keep going? What can I control?" Focusing on these things gave me a place to stand and move forward from. It didn't magically eliminate my feelings of disappointment, but it started to get me unstuck and fueled hope once again.

I controlled the ability to write another blog post, ride my recumbent bike for twenty minutes a day, do my exercises, initiate contact with friends, choose an optimistic attitude, eat right, and not watch TV during the day. When I added a pound of control, I was following the advice of Theodore Roosevelt, who said, "Do what you can with what you have where you are."

Marilu Henner said, "Being in control of your life and having realistic expectations about your day-to-day challenges are the keys to stress management, which is perhaps the most important ingredient to living a happy, healthy, and rewarding life."

Ingredient #3: A pinch of suffering

I learned to expect suffering. If our worldview does not include the possibility of heartache and pain, our expectations will not be met. I didn't go looking for pain, but I learned to accept that suffering will be a normal part of my human experience for as long as I live on earth. Expecting a struggle will soften the blow of disappointment. C.S. Lewis learned this firsthand: "We were promised sufferings. They were part of the program. We were even told, 'Blessed are they that mourn,' and I accept it. I've got nothing that I hadn't bargained for." Theodore Rubin said, "The problem is not that there are problems. The problem is expecting otherwise and thinking that having problems is a problem."

I realized that if I didn't like my circumstances, I didn't need to change my circumstances as much as I needed to change the way I looked at my circumstances. A pity party is a lonely party no one wants to come to. Accepting hardship opened the door to resources I hadn't known existed when I had been focused solely on how unfair my life had become.

Beating the greener grass syndrome

The ability to set realistic expectations is often impacted by "the greener grass syndrome." That syndrome says, "The grass is greener on the other side of the fence" or "Things are better anywhere but here." If we are suffering from this syndrome, we expect and believe circumstances, opportunities, experiences, and conditions are much better somewhere else.

I suffered with this syndrome. Once, while I was riding a stationary bike in a fitness club, a triathlon was in progress on several of the TV screens overhead. I got excited as I watched the contestants ride their bikes at top speed around the course. As they pedaled, I pedaled even harder on the bike I was riding. When they transitioned to the running phase, however, I felt a surge of envy rise within me. I said to myself, "I sure wish I could run. It's not fair that I can't." I envied those runners and their ability to run. I envied them because I had loved running when I had been able to run. I had loved the thrill of competition and achieving personal best times because of my training and hard work.

To be honest, I was shocked I had these feelings of envy. I had dealt with the loss of my running already—or so I thought. It shows how important it is to not only set realistic expectations but to also hold on to them tightly.

The good news was that I caught myself turning green with envy quickly, drank from the cup of honesty, grabbed hold of what I could control, embraced my suffering, and accepted it all as part of the normal process of recovery. I eventually turned my envy into gratitude for the ability to cycle and stay active riding a stationary bike.

I even developed several strategies for beating the greener grass syndrome.

1. Stop looking over the fence.

It's not about whether you look over the fence or not — of course, you will. The key is what to do after you realize you're looking. Will you choose to turn away from your self-defeating, negative thoughts or fixate on them? If you fixate on them, your own grass will turn brown, and you'll stay stuck. If you choose to turn away, you will be able to find gratitude and happiness where you are. True happiness starts in your mind. Dale Carnegie advised, "It isn't what you have or who you are or where you are or what you are doing that makes you happy or unhappy. It is what you think about it."

2. Stop bitterness from taking root.

One of the ditches you can fall into when disappointed by unmet expectations is bitterness. Bitterness forms when a hurt or an offense is held onto and not released. Bitterness is released by forgiveness — when you no longer want the person who hurt you to hurt because of what happened to you. Solomon in his wisdom said, "A heart at peace gives life to the body, but envy rots the bones."[43] Ron McManus said, "Bitterness is like drinking poison and waiting for the other person to die."

3. Accept your limitations.

Accepting limitations opens the door to finding realistic expectations. Accepting your current reality opens your eyes to see what you have to work with. Those in the counseling profession spend a lot of time helping clients re-orient themselves to deal with the life they have instead of the life they expected to have. It may seem deflating initially, but when the adjustment is made, the rebuilding process begins.

4. Study yourself to see what you have to work with.

What do you have to work with? What's in your toolbox? What talent, under-developed skill, hidden gift, or ability is in your hand that you can use? If you can't run, what can you do? If you can't work in the same job as before, what can you do now? Frederick Keonig said, "We tend to forget that happiness doesn't come as a result of getting something we don't have, but rather of recognizing and appreciating what we do have."

5. Step into the opportunities you have.

As things change, new opportunities open up. The key is to prepare yourself so that when the new opportunities come, you're not so busy looking at the grass on the other side of the fence that you don't notice them. The door to mountain biking opened for me after the door to running closed. Alexander Graham Bell said, "When one door closes, another door opens; but we so often look so long and so regretfully upon the closed door, that we do not see the ones which open for us."

Final thought

If you follow the above recipe and strategy for dealing with expectations, the grass will be greener on your side of the fence — because you will have spent your time and energy watering, nurturing, and fertilizing it!

Detour Reflections

❖ What unrealistic expectations do you need to lay down so you can pick up realistic expectations?

❖ Of the five strategies for beating the greener grass syndrome, which one do you need to apply to your situation?

Chapter 17: Waiting

Waiting is exhausting and not an activity I was keen on embracing. I'm a man of action, and I like to make things happen, not wait for things to happen. Unfortunately, on my detour, I didn't have a choice. I had to learn how to wait when the days turned into weeks, the weeks turned into months, and the months turned into years.

But I knew that I was not alone in my waiting. As Dr, Seuss wrote, "Everyone is just waiting."[44]

Waiting, on one level, is "remaining inactive in one place while expecting something." On another level, it has the potential to be an opportunity. When it came to waiting, I refused to settle for Voltaire's pessimism that said, "We never live; we are always in the expectation of living." My approach was to find a better way to wait, and to help in this process I asked two questions: 1) How can waiting be more than passive inactivity? and 2) How can I be fully alive while waiting?

Waiting as more than passive inactivity

To move past the passive inactivity of waiting, you have to come to terms, first of all, with the reality of your situation. You can't change your position if you are unaware of your starting point. While I waited on one occasion, I tried my hand at poetry to describe my waiting. The poem was simply called "Waiting."

Waiting comes in all shapes and sizes
And is not without its dips and surprises —
Waiting for blood work to go in the right direction,
Waiting for an end to this nasty infection,
Waiting to get off this oxy dependence,
Waiting with patience for help from the Transcendent,
Waiting for physio to start up again,
Waiting for the painful stretching to come to an end,

Waiting to go back for surgery again,
Waiting for the swelling and pain to end.
Waiting to walk takes such a long while.
Waiting to drive resembled walking the extra mile.
Waiting to work went on for such a long time
And forced me to dance a new rhythm and rhyme.

The key to waiting

While I was waiting for the detour to end, so many things were outside my control. Over and over again I had to accept my situation and ride out the storm I was going through. On the flip side, there was one thing I could control—the way I chose to look at things.

I had control over which perspective I would look at my life from. If I had watched and waited from the dark and unattractive underbelly of passive resentment, I would have missed the chance to learn, find new life, and receive new strength. It took discipline and a willingness to fire up my imagination, but the new view I gained from the effort was worth it.

The windows I looked through while waiting

During my waiting, I looked through several windows which fired up my imagination and opened up my heart and mind to fresh, life-giving perspectives.

- **I tried wondering while waiting.**

While I waited, I reflected on the gifts I had been given, the talents I possessed, the gratitude I wanted to express, and the people who gave their best. This left me feeling blessed.

- **I tried wandering while waiting.**

One of the activities I practiced while waiting was to smell the flowers while riding my electric scooter around the neighborhood. I talked to neighbors. One neighbor who stood out was the one with Parkinson's disease. In getting to know his story, I discovered that his burden was much greater than mine. I also wandered through the pages of inspiring stories of people who had overcome adversity in heroic ways.

- **I tried weeping while waiting.**

My pain and hurt needed a relief valve. During my waiting, that valve often took the form of tears. In the weeping I found healing and a release of pent-up pain and emotion. In order to heal, you have to weep, and the time spent waiting is an opportune time to do just that.

- **I tried waltzing while waiting.**

Waiting offered me an opportunity to learn new "dance steps" — new ways of acting and reacting in certain situations. People I had been impatient with in the past were now the same people I learned to understand and accept. Waiting showed me ways to be a better person.

- **I tried widening my view while waiting.**

Waiting gave me time to explore new worlds that were within my reach. I developed new eyes to see the suffering of others and grew new muscles of empathy.

- **I tried being wrecked while waiting.**

I learned that being wrecked can lead to old, unworkable priorities and patterns being destroyed. Waiting disturbed my status quo and left me changed for the better.

Learning to sing *Dayenu*

It's hard to wait and not have moments when you wish things were different. This was true for me, and it was also true for the Jews. To help them wait, they sang a song that helped them deal with their waiting. The song, called *"Dayenu,"*[45] is sung during the Passover holiday and means, "It would have been enough for us." It expresses gratitude to God for what he has done and fosters contentment and a thankful spirit. The middle section (based on Israel's story) goes something like this:

If He had split the sea for us — it would have been enough.
If He had led us through on dry land — it would have been enough.
If He had drowned our oppressors — it would have been enough.
If He had provided for our needs in the wilderness for forty years — it would have been enough.
If He had fed us manna — it would have been enough.

My *dayenu* moment happened one day while the sun was shining. Because the rain had stopped, I could go for a scooter ride through the woods near our house. While on the ride, I met a friend who also rides a scooter. I call him a friend because I have talked to him numerous times and know him by name. He is probably in his seventies and struggles with the later stages of Parkinson's disease. On this particular day, I parked beside him, and we had a long conversation. He was recovering from an operation to replace a battery in a device in his chest that helps regulate his out-of-control muscles. He described the disease in detail. He had been diagnosed eighteen years earlier and realized he might not have many years left to live. As I listened to his story, I thought of my situation and felt a surge of gratitude to God for what he had done for me up to that point. I said to myself: "What I have in my hand right now is enough!" I sang this song on that day:

I have a scooter to ride on — it is enough.
I have a beating heart, eyes, ears, mind, taste buds — it is enough.
I have a roof over my head and clean water to drink — it is enough.
I have a laptop to type on and a mind to direct my fingers — it is enough.
I have a loving wife who drives me around and feeds me well — it is enough.
I have money to pay the bills and provide for our daily needs — it is enough.

I have friends who call and come to visit—it is enough.

I can walk with the help of crutches and a walker—it is enough.

I have a physiotherapist helping me prepare to walk again—it is enough.

I have books to read, podcasts to listen to, and hockey to watch—it is enough.

I have a church community of friends to grow spiritually with—it is enough.

I could have focused on what was missing that day, but, because of my friend, I chose to look at what I held in my hand and say, "*Dayenu*—what I have is enough!"

The land between

Waiting puts us in the "land between." The "land between" is the place of transition between two phases of life. It is the journey from life as it was to life as it will be. The "land between" is a time to reflect on the past, and it is an opportunity to develop new skills for the future. The "land between" is a time to accept the uncontrollable nature of life. The "land between" resembles a wasteland, a desert place between the old and the new.

The biggest challenge in the "land between" is to not waste the opportunities it presents—for personal growth, deep change, and purposeful living. Many people miss these opportunities because they have chosen to spend this time wallowing in self-pity, regret, and complaining. That was true for the Israelites on their journey between Egypt and the Promised Land. They spent far too much time grumbling and complaining about how life was unfair and how God had abandoned them in the desert. Their spirit of impatience resulted in more pain and an even longer journey in the "land between."

As I learned to slow down and mine the "land between" for gold and valuable gems, I made all kinds of discoveries. I discovered freedom to let go of my need to control. I met new people and formed lasting friendships. I learned new skills and developed some of my untapped potential. I increased my ability to trust in God to lead me when I couldn't see where I was going. I gained a fresh appreciation for the value of community. I was given time to volunteer on projects I had previously been too busy for.

A prayer while you wait

I end this chapter on waiting with the following prayer:

> May God visit you with patience in your season of waiting. May the barren landscape of your adversity become the fertile soil of new growth. May the God of grace revive your spirit and give you back your laughter. May you find God with you in your pain and trustworthy as you wait. May the one who restores what's been taken, meet you in the desert and journey with you to the other side. Amen.[46]

Detour Reflections

❖ What are you waiting for?

❖ How does your perspective need to change so your waiting can be life-giving?

Chapter 18: Fellowship

Fellowship is defined in several ways. It describes, on the one hand, "a friendly relationship among people" or "a group of people who have similar interests." On the other hand, it is the English word used to translate the Greek word *koinonia,* meaning "communion, joint participation; the share which one has in anything."[47] During recovery, I experienced both kinds of fellowship. I had friendly relationships with some people and met others who had similar interests, but I also encountered some who were joint participants in what I was experiencing. The second group were a life saver.

Fellowship during my detour became so much more than the fellowship I remember growing up. Fellowship growing up was the word we used to describe the potluck meals we had downstairs after church. We drank Kool-aid, talked about the weather, and ate casseroles together. Detour fellowship was about connection, togetherness, partnership, and the sharing of life in depth. In comparison, potlucks were skin-deep fellowship.

A powerful picture of fellowship

The fellowship I experienced during the detour was like a tent peg in a windstorm. The best way to explain the fellowship I experienced is to use some illustrations from a favorite story of mine, J.R.R. Tolkien's series of books, *The Lord of the Rings.* The main character, Frodo, was given the responsibility to carry a powerful ring over treacherous terrain to Mordor and destroy the ring there.

The success of Frodo's journey would rest in large part on the help of a group of friends called "the fellowship of the ring." These traveling companions were not allowed to carry the ring directly but were called upon to support Frodo as he carried it. There is a scene near the end of the journey that captures the essence of fellowship. When a character named Sam saw Frodo collapse under the weight of the ring's burden, Sam instantly picked Frodo up in his arms and said, "Frodo, I may not be able to carry the ring, but I can carry you!"

Earlier on his journey, Frodo questioned why he was the one burdened with responsibility for the ring, saying, "I wish it need not have happened in my time." His wise friend Gandalf replied, "So do I, and so do all who live to see such times. But that is not for them to decide. All we have to decide is what to do with the time that is given us."

My fellowship carried me

There was a long list of people who helped me weather the storms and fight the battles I couldn't fight on my own. None of them could take my suffering away and carry it themselves because that was mine to carry. What they could do was take the journey with me and carry me as I carried my burden. Their practical and helpful actions included the following:

- My fellowship showed up and sat with me without feeling the need to say anything.
- My fellowship sent emails and texts to remind me they were thinking of me and praying for me.
- My fellowship picked up the phone and called to chat for a few brief minutes at just the right times.
- My fellowship shared their own pain with me as a means of being real and authentic.
- My fellowship shared their pleasures with me so I could celebrate with them.
- My fellowship allowed me to help them by giving advice, buying them lunch, and offering a prayer.
- My fellowship cried with me or let me cry with them without me feeling the need to squelch my tears.
- My fellowship laughed with me by sharing a video or funny story.
- My fellowship took the initiative to do the chores I couldn't do.

Fellowship as standing alone together

Two ingredients you need to survive and thrive during times of adversity are internal strength of character and a band of brothers and sisters standing with you.

The first paratroopers in the US Army, called Easy Company, had these two ingredients. One of the company's regular training drills was to run up and down a three-mile hill called *Currahee*, which means, "We stand alone together." The hill became a symbol of the deep bond forged between the soldiers as they prepared for the D-Day invasion of Normandy and the battles that followed. Each paratrooper did stand alone at the airplane door before jumping, but once the battle began, they lived and fought together. It was said that "They depended on each other, and the world depended on them."

Standing alone for me was the experience of pain, immobility, loss, and lack of purpose that followed the accident. But deep bonds of fellowship were forged as I let go of my need to be the hero and fight my battles alone. In humility, I let others help me when I couldn't help myself. I spoke words of appreciation to those who helped, and I gave myself permission to find safe people I could share my pain with. As a result, I experienced the strength and healing that came through the prayers of others.

A lesson from African culture

One of the strengths of African culture is the value that is placed on community. In the West, we sometimes put the good of the individual ahead of the good of the community — to our detriment. African church leader Desmond Tutu said, "You can't exist as a human being in isolation." A word that captures this idea is the term *Ubuntu*.[48] The term first appeared as an idea in South African society in the mid-19th century. At first, it was translated as "human nature, humanness, humanity; virtue, goodness, roughness." It later grew to be a term used by religious, political, and community leaders in various settings. Here are some of the ways *Ubuntu* was understood:

- "A person with *Ubuntu* is open and available to others, affirming of others, does not feel threatened that others are able and good, based from a proper self-assurance that comes from knowing that he or she belongs in a greater whole and is diminished when others are humiliated or diminished, when others are tortured or oppressed." – Desmond Tutu
- "It speaks about our interconnectedness. You can't be human all by yourself, and when you have this quality – *Ubuntu* – you are known for your generosity." – Desmond Tutu
- "A traveler through a country would stop at a village and he didn't have to ask for food or for water. Once he stops, the people give him food and attend him. That is one aspect of *Ubuntu*, but it will have various aspects. *Ubuntu* does not mean that people should not enrich themselves. The question therefore is: Are you going to do so in order to enable the community around you to be able to improve?" – Nelson Mandela

Integrating *Ubuntu* with fellowship

Learning about *Ubuntu* challenged me to look out for the impact of the community around me. Even though perseverance and individual effort were essential for me to push through the pain and make strides in my recovery, there was much more going on around me that I needed to pay attention to. Here are three lessons I learned from *Ubuntu*.

- **Remind yourself often that "It's not just about me."**

It is natural to be self-absorbed when you are hurting, but if that attitude continues for too long, it turns unhealthy. *Ubuntu* says, "It's not all about me; it's also about you. Who are the people who need me to care for them? Who needs to be thanked? Who needs my listening ear? I'm never completely alone, for God is always with me. My community needs me to give something back in order for it to be all it can be."

- **Take time for solitude, but don't isolate yourself.**

When I was struggling through surgeries, rehabilitation, and adversity, it was easy for me to turn inward and feel unable to reach out and connect to others. The problem was that this left me isolated. The solution was to take time for solitude (where I practiced spiritual reading, journaling, reflection, and prayer) but to also intentionally reach out to others and initiate connection.

- **Remain open and generous with others.**

Staying connected with others requires a willingness to share joys and struggles in meaningful ways. I was thrilled the day I was given the green light by my physiotherapist to ride a "real" bike outside after three years of waiting. This milestone was not reached simply because of my rugged individual effort. It was reached because I had a community of committed people who cheered me on and invested in my life so it could happen. When I told people, "I rode a bike outside today," tears welled up inside me, and the news brought fresh air to those who had helped me get there.

A tribute to my fellowship

There is a long list of those in my fellowship who walked beside me and made up my community. The choir of cheerleaders was made up of both professionals and amateurs. Yes, I had to carry the suffering, but I didn't have to do it alone. My fellowship included:
- God (the Father, Son, and Holy Spirit)
- doctors (orthopedic surgeons, GPs, hospital staff members, infectious disease specialists)
- nurses (in the operating room, on the ward, in the intensive care unit, in my home)
- paramedics (helicopter pilots, volunteer firefighters, ambulance drivers)
- physiotherapists (in the hospital, in my home, in the clinic)

- home care workers (for food prep, cleaning, personal care — and even a podiatrist)
- occupational therapists
- counsellors
- lawyers
- insurance specialists
- mentors (those who modeled the way)
- enduring individuals (friends and family who never gave up)
- authors (who wrote the stories that inspired me and fanned hope)

A final thought

If you try to go it alone — hold everything in, don't ask for help, keep the pain inside, don't share your story, hold on to your hurt, and believe no one understands or cares — things will get worse.

If you go on the journey with others — ask for help, let other survivors tell you their stories, let go of your bitterness by confessing it to others, offer forgiveness, seek counsel, admit that you can't do it on your own, get honest with how you feel, and commit to doing things differently — you will get better.

Detour Reflections

❖ When have you experienced a fellowship of support during a time of suffering or loss?

❖ Who are the people in your fellowship who need to be appreciated for the support they've been for you? Now, go and express your thanks.

Chapter 19: Discipline

Discipline for many people is a dirty word. It carries with it the connotation of hard work, correction, repetitive action, sweat, waking up to an alarm clock, and doing what you don't want to do so you can have what you really want. Sir Winston Churchill once said, "It's not good enough to do our best. Sometimes we have to do what is required." That takes discipline.

Discipline during the detour was one of the ways I stayed anchored and grounded so I wouldn't blow away in the wind. Discipline did include the elements listed above, but, instead of being a dirty word, it became the handle I held on to as I climbed out of my predicament toward recovery.

What discipline is

By definition, discipline includes such concepts as training and conditions imposed for the improvement of physical powers.[49] While on recovery's road, the conditions I imposed on myself and the training I participated in made improvement in all areas of my life possible. Discipline not only improved my physical powers but also my spiritual resilience, self-control, and sense of hope and optimism. Discipline was not the change itself but the road I traveled in order to make the changes.

My discipline needed an underlying "Why am I doing this?" in order for me to stay motivated so "What on earth am I doing?" did not bring my training to a standstill. My answer to the "Why am I doing this?" question went something like this: "I want to live out my purpose of helping as many people as possible, which will only be accomplished if I am in the best physical, emotional, spiritual, and intellectual shape I can be."

Disciplines that take you where you want to go

This list is by no means exhaustive but is just a sample of some of the core disciplines that helped me climb toward recovery and grow during the detour.

1. The discipline of positive belief

Nurturing a positive belief is something I had to work on every day and can be compared to what happens when a person lifts weights. When we lift weights, the extra strain on our muscles tears down the old muscles and makes way for the building of new and stronger muscles. Building a positive belief is a process of tearing down limiting and ineffective beliefs in order to make room for new and stronger beliefs.

The discipline of positive belief helps us to stop living in the land of regret and "if only" and moves us to the land "How will I?" Negative beliefs keep us down, while positive beliefs fuel creativity and productive action. The discipline of positive belief is a conscious choice to not be preoccupied with limitations but to look instead at the opportunities that are right in front of us.

A negative attitude says, "Poor me, I can't walk more than a block. Poor me, I have another surgery coming up. Poor me, I went on a road trip and couldn't go for a hike. Poor me, I can only work for three months, and then I have to stop again."

A positive attitude says, "I'm so excited because I got to ride a three-wheeled bike on the sandy shore of the Oregon coast! I'm so excited because I was able to drive and enjoy amazing scenery on our road trip last weekend. I'm so excited because I have a window in time when I can connect with people, do what I love, and anticipate my next surgery, which will only enhance the quality of my life."

2. The discipline of remembering

Another way I trained myself to be strong in spirit, mind, and body was to remember traumatic events. Studies prove there is value in remembering traumatic events, but because it is hard work, it requires discipline to do. These events could be the death of a loved one, the day the house burned down, the day the soldiers died, or the day the road you were on ended.

"Remember" comes from two words: "re," which means "again," and "memor," which means "mindful."[50] I chose to be "mindful again" of our motorcycle accident. My wife and I went back to the crash site more than once to bring to mind again what had happened on that stretch of highway in 2011. We call the anniversary date of the accident our "crashiversary," which is a way to remember yet move forward.

Remembering bad events is more helpful than forgetting them, according to Dr. Alan Manevitz, a psychiatrist at New York's Lenox Hill Hospital who worked with victims of 9/11. [51] When remembering triggers trauma, it creates a doorway into deeper healing and can push people to get more help with their loss.

Remembering reminds us of what we have, not just what we have lost. As I remembered the events of my loss, I was able to arrive at a place of gratitude for what I had left and experience greater strength and readiness to embrace my new normal.

Remembering encourages others, who are going through a similar situation, to persevere and not give up.

Remembering integrates our traumatic experiences with everyday life. If we don't find space for difficult events in our memories, they hold us back and keep us from moving forward to a place of healing.

3. The discipline of journaling

Another discipline that helps process trauma, pain, and adversity is journaling. I had practiced journaling prior to the accident, but while I was on my detour, journaling took on new meaning. My journaling efforts started out sporadically in the early days after the accident due to the pain I was experiencing and the fact that my writing arm was broken. Eventually, however, I began to journal regularly.

Journaling has many forms. We can write on paper or record things electronically. We can use journaling to record events, catalog quotes and wise sayings, draw pictures, write out prayers, do personal planning, and express our creativity.

Journaling provides a structure for processing life events and emotions, increases self-awareness, and offers a way to see things from a fresh perspective. Journaling gives us the opportunity to think more clearly as we put our thoughts and feelings down on paper. I agree with what Henry Ford said: "Thinking is hard work. That's why so few people do it."

Journaling impacted my life in numerous ways. It provided a record I used to encourage myself days later. It helped me release pent-up emotions (anger, frustration, stress, doubt, and fear). It helped me detach from past events and paved the way for healthier self-talk and the neutralizing of self-sabotaging conversations.

Journaling reinforced what I was learning and increased retention of what I was hearing or reading. It reminded me of my values, which anchored me when I was under stress. It helped me see options I hadn't seen until I started writing. It promoted honesty and cut through denial and self-deception. Journaling created a space to listen to the voice of wisdom and the voice of God.

Journaling provided a place for me to rediscover purpose and find an answer to "What's next?" Journaling developed the writer within me. It gave me a way to track improvement and visualize personal progress. It created a fun yet safe place to express wild and crazy ideas. I didn't always want to journal, but, like any discipline, when I simply did it, the benefits followed.

4. The discipline of action

Action may not sound like a discipline, but I am suggesting it is. The reason action is a discipline is that, without it, we do not get to where we need to go—both inside and out. The opposite of action is procrastination and inaction, which kill good intentions and hinder healthy recovery. Action runs counter to the voice inside our head that whispers all kinds of reasons why we can't do what we should be doing or why we'd be better off waiting just one more day before getting into gear.

What barriers hold action back? Here were a few of mine. Fear held me back from action, saying, "I'm afraid I might fail." Doubt said, "I'm not sure I can do this!" Anxiety said, "I'm worried about what might happen if I step out." Apathy whispered, "I don't really care what happens." Pessimism said, "It's no use, since it won't work out anyway." Ignorance said, "I don't know where to start."

When I was curtailed from normal activities, it would have been easy for me to resign myself to inactivity while I waited to heal. If I had allowed myself to get bogged down in the emotional malaise of waiting, I would have sunk into an even deeper place of melancholy and frustration. There was a need for a time to rest, sleep, and be with my pain and difficulty, but I came to realize I couldn't wait for all the outside factors to be right before I entered the arena of action.

There were five principles I followed to help me move into the discipline of action:

- First, I had to figure out what would make my life worthwhile. I had to discover my purpose. I had to get a grip on why I was on the earth.
- Second, I had to move my purpose into goals to achieve or problems to solve.
- Third, I had to figure out all the necessary steps I needed to take to accomplish my goals or solve my problems.
- Fourth, I had to turn my action steps into a daily action list. One simple system I used during the detour was to write out the half dozen things I needed to do that day on a three by five card and carry it around with me until everything on the list was done.
- Fifth, I had to celebrate the small wins. "Things that get rewarded get repeated." I knew that if I celebrated the actions that moved me towards my purpose and goals, I'd keep doing more of them.

5. The discipline of baby steps

For over sixteen months, I was not allowed to put any weight on my right leg. At one point, the surgery on my right leg was so radical that I couldn't even touch the ground with my toe. This meant I had to climb stairs on one leg, one crutch, and a handrail.

The discipline I practiced to learn this new skill was the discipline of baby steps. I wouldn't be allowed to go home until I could climb stairs the new way. The fourteen steps that I had to climb to get into my house waited for me. I needed to take the baby steps required to conquer the makeshift staircase in the hospital hallway before I could go home. My first attempt to climb the practice stairs was a total failure. The physiotherapist was kind and encouraging, but the steps were too high, and I was too scared.

When I came back the next day, I discovered there were steps half the size on the other side of the staircase. This allowed me to take the baby steps I needed to learn this new skill. I succeeded on my first attempt and returned to my hospital room victorious. The next day, I went back to the full-sized steps—and guess what? I climbed them as well. Baby steps allowed my confidence and competence to grow, slowly but surely.

Final Thought

I end this chapter with a few wise words from Jim Rohn: "We must all suffer one of two things: the pain of discipline or the pain of regret. Discipline is the bridge between goals and accomplishment. Success is nothing more than a few simple disciplines, practiced every day."

Detour Reflections

❖ What is the "why" in your life that motivates you to walk discipline's pathway?

❖ Which of the five disciplines best describes where you need to focus your efforts right now?

Chapter 20: Healing

Healing can be quick and easy if the injury or hurt is small. However, if the hurt is deep and the injury complicated, healing can require a long and painful process before we finally arrive at a place of wholeness. Complete and final healing is reserved for heaven, but thankfully we can experience moments of wholeness here on earth.

Care and cure

A distinction that helped me understand the healing journey was to see the synergy between care and cure. Henri Nouwen describes the interplay this way:

> Care is something other than cure. Cure means "change." A doctor, a lawyer, a minister, a social worker — they all want to use their professional skills to bring about changes in people's lives. They get paid for whatever kind of cure they can bring about. But cure, desirable as it may be, can easily become violent, manipulative, and even destructive if it does not grow out of care. Care is being with, crying out with, suffering with, feeling with. Care is compassion. It is claiming the truth that the other person is my brother or sister, human, mortal, vulnerable, like I am...When care is our first concern, cure can be received as a gift. Often we are not able to cure, but we are always able to care. To care is to be human.[52]

Care can be defined as to show concern, to demonstrate compassion, to give attention to, to meet the needs of another person in a loving way. Cure is defined as "restoration of health; recovery from disease; a method or course of medical treatment used to restore health; an agent, such as a drug, that restores health; a remedy."[53]

133

Cure without care may provide the best medicine and treatment available but leave you feeling isolated and angry, with no one willing to listen to your story. Cure without care may use the latest technology to grow a new bone in your leg but leave you with nobody to comfort and cheer you on through the pain and effort necessary to complete the healing.

Care can be offered by a loving family and supportive friends, but, without proper medical treatment, it will not mend your broken body. Care without cure can offer optimism but no pathway to kill the raging infection or mend torn tendons.

Care without cure is like sleeping on a soft pillow top mattress with no supporting box spring. Cure without care is like sleeping on a sheet of plywood that provides support but no comfort.

Thankfully, I had both care and cure and witnessed firsthand the dynamic relationship between care and cure. I had ten surgeries and numerous other treatments, but the cure was matched by the loving care of a whole team of people who walked with me towards wholeness.

Six qualities needed to heal

Healing is not automatic or guaranteed in this life. Some people die, get worse, or are left with chronic pain that stays with them throughout life. Healing is a complicated subject. What I found from my own experience and my research was that where healing is possible, certain qualities enhance the depth, speed, and extent of the healing. We are emotional, intellectual, and spiritual beings, so even when we are left with physical deficits that are not healed, there is a great deal of healing work that can still be done. My healing went deep, yet I was still left with physical limitations I'll have for the rest of my life. To get to where I finally ended up, I embraced these six qualities and found they were critical to my healing journey.

1. **Admit you are broken.**

This sounds easier than it seems. I've seen people find so much comfort in their suffering that they don't really want to get well. Their pain becomes their identity and denial their comfort. Healing requires honesty.

2. **Be ready for healing.**

When healing requires a painful cure, you need to be ready to embrace the cure. The journey between brokenness and healing is a painful one. Whenever I had another surgery looming, I dreaded it and struggled with "surgery fatigue" (a term I made up and found useful). Deep down, however, I knew that if I wanted to get well, I had to face the pain head on.

3. **Be open to receive help from others.**

I found it easy to receive help from my surgeon because I trusted him (and perhaps because he mostly worked on me while I was asleep). I was more guarded when the psychologist helped me deal with my emotional pain. I did embrace his help eventually because I wanted the healing more than I wanted to feel safe.

4. **Be willing to forgive those who have caused or allowed the brokenness.**

I had to forgive the driver who pulled out in front of us. I had to work through the "Why me?" questions and let God be God instead of blaming him for letting something bad happen. When I forgave the driver and gave God permission to work some good out of this bad event, the door to healing opened up.

5. **Practice patience and courage.**

Patience was in short supply when the road ended and the detour became my reality. Over time, however, I realized that without patience and the courage to press on, the healing process would slow to a crawl. Patience and courage grew one breath and one decision at a time.

6. Invite God on the healing journey.

As soon as I woke up in the intensive care unit, I started talking to God. I didn't always have happy thoughts towards him, but from the start I invited him to go with me on this healing journey. I don't understand why God chooses to heal some but not others. While living with this tension, I trust his wisdom. I am grateful for the healing I experienced, but I keep in my mind the fact that none of us will get off this planet alive.

Final thought

Healing can be messy and emotional. It can also take more time than you expect. The three times I came off oxycodone (an effective but highly addictive pain killer), the healing process worked differently each time. The third time I came off the drug, I had more of the qualities needed to heal. The first time, I didn't utilize my doctor's support and struggled with seven days of sleepless nights and intense agitation. The third time, I took my doctor's support to heart. He told me to take more time and reduce the dosage gradually. I also had more courage and the belief that healing would come in time.

Detour Reflections

❖ When have you been broken? What have you done to move from brokenness to a place of healing?

❖ What advice would you give to someone facing the uphill climb of recovery and healing?

Detour in Pictures

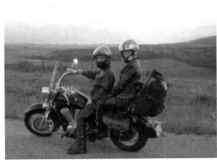

Vicky and I on one of our many bike trips.

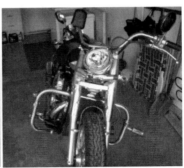

Our Honda Shadow 750 after April 23, 2011.

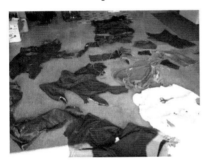

At the scene, all of our clothes were cut off.

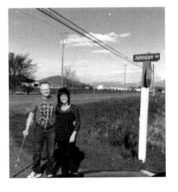

We went back to the accident scene two years later.

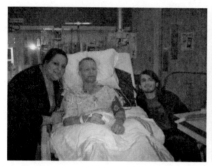

Our kids, Elena and Caleb, by my side in the ICU at RCH.

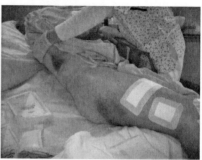

Most of my injuries were on the right side.

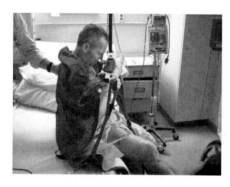

A hospital lift got me moving again.

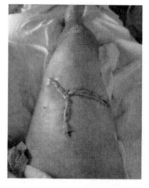

After surgery number one, the view was shocking.

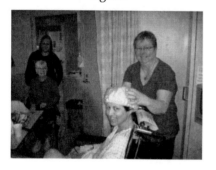

Debbie washed Vicky's hair without any water.

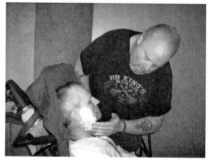

Rob gave me my first shave.

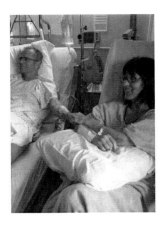

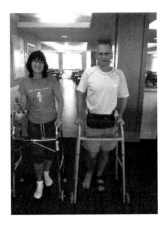

Vicky and I were together for 10 days at RCH.

Walking with walkers together.

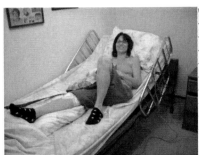

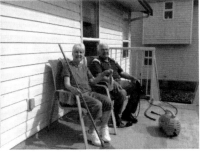

Vicky lived with her parents until I came home.

Vicky's Mom and Dad helped in so many ways!

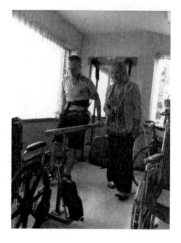

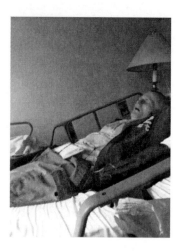

One of my physio workouts in the early days.

I spent a lot of time doing this.

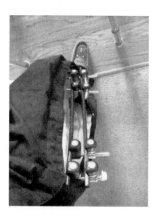

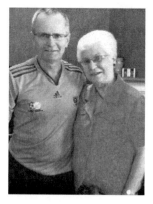

On day 201, six inches of my right femur were cut out, and a fixator was attached.

My mom was by my side as often as she could be.

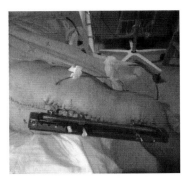

On day 375, the bone transporter went on my leg to facilitate new bone growth.

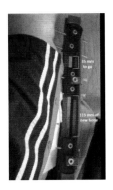

The bone transporter, well on its way to finishing the job.

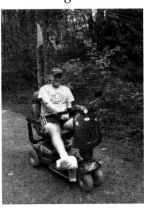

When I needed to get outside, this was my ride for two years.

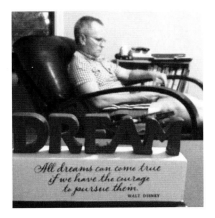

I spent over 5,000 hours in the recliner but had purpose.

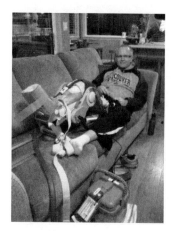

Day 1006: the continuous passive motion machine helped keep my knee bending 24/7.

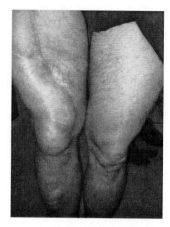

This is what my legs look like now.

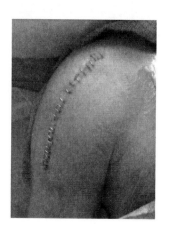

My tenth and final surgery removed the hardware from my right arm.

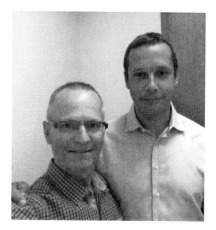

I stand beside my skilled orthopedic surgeon, Dr. Darius Viskontas.

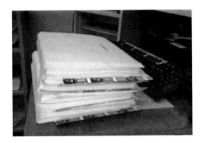

The hospital files added up.

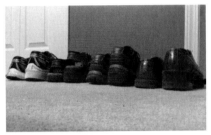

I have lifts to make up for the 2 ½-inch difference in leg length.

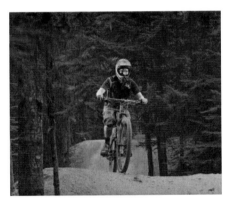

Here I am mountain biking at Whistler's Bike Park in 2016.

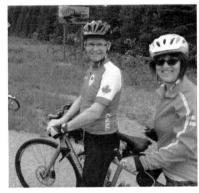

Vicky and I on a 600 kilometer tandem bike ride in 2016.

Part 3: The Road Begins Again

There comes a time in every detour when we finally make our way back onto the main road. The transition isn't always smooth and seamless but can often include bumps, disorientation, adjustments, and uneasiness.

This part of my story is about the challenges I experienced when integrating my new normal into the life I had once known. In the novel *The Lord of the Rings*, the character Frodo had to make a similar transition after he returned from his epic journey. He came back to the Shire (his old life) and found that it had stayed the same — but he himself had changed. As a result, the re-engagement was challenging.

Getting back on the road again after my detour was a challenging transition for me. It involved merging the events and lessons I had learned on my detour with the ordinary world I had left behind. The world I was returning to was very similar to what it had been, but I had changed.

In Part 3, I tackle several themes, including work, mindset, resistance, momentum, brokenness, and impact. Re-entry was much harder than I thought it would be, but I pressed on in hope and faced each challenge head on.

Chapter 21: Preparation

Abraham Lincoln once said, "Give me six hours to chop down a tree, and I will spend the first four sharpening the ax." This is a metaphor illustrating the impact preparation has in our lives. The better prepared we are for what lies ahead, the better. No one knows exactly what is ahead, but I can say with 100 percent certainty that the day will come when you will be called upon to deal with a detour of some kind. That experience will test your mettle and reveal the quality of your preparation.

In reality, we are always preparing, but there are certain principles and practices that will make us better prepared for whatever comes in life. Once I was on my detour, I realized that I already had several habits, practices, and ways of thinking that served me well. The key question I attempt to answer in this chapter is: "What does it look like to be prepared for the challenges that come into our lives?"

The story of two explorers

In October 1911, two teams made their final preparations for their attempts to be the first explorers to reach the South Pole.[54] One team, led by Roald Amundsen, raced to victory and returned home safely. The other team, led by Robert Falcon Scott, reached the Pole thirty-four days later and all died on the return trip.

What was the difference? Preparation. Amundsen believed that you don't wait until you're in an unexpected storm to discover that you need more strength and endurance—you prepare ahead of time. He and his team lived with Inuit and learned how to dress, live, and survive in freezing temperatures. He became an expert dog handler, ate raw dolphin, and became a skilled skier. He took more supplies than he needed and used black flags to carefully mark his route on the way to the Pole in case of bad weather on his return.

Robert Falcon Scott, on the other hand, did not train properly for his expedition. He relied on the knowledge he already had and failed to learn from those who had lived in similar conditions. Instead of dogs, he chose ponies, which didn't hold up in the cold. He took untested motor sledges, which broke down under the extreme conditions. He took just enough supplies and didn't mark his return route. The rest is history.

Behaviors of the prepared

The stories of Amundsen and Scott teach several lessons that reinforce the need to make preparation a daily habit and part of the fabric of life.

- **Learn from and hang out with wise people.**

Amundsen lived with and learned from the Inuit, who had a proven track record of survival in harsh conditions.

For years, I have made it a habit to learn from historical mentors—to read their stories, learn their wisdom, and be guided by their insights. I've gained wisdom from family members, friends, coaches, leaders, and others. They have helped me to be prepared to live and thrive under difficult circumstances.

- **Temper optimism with a good dose of realism.**

Untempered optimism clouds our ability to accept the possibility of trouble. Scott's optimism cost him his life and the lives of his teammates because he had not planned for the possibility of "bad luck" on the trip home. Amundsen hoped for good weather but stored food and built in a safety margin in case there were storms.

During my detour and re-entry into normal life, I continually hoped for better days, but I braced myself for challenges and unexpected outcomes. I prepared for the down days and was not surprised when setbacks came my way.

- **Practice hardship before you have to.**

Amundsen trained himself so his mind ran his body. He practiced enduring hardship before he was on the actual trip. This prepared him to endure hardship when he was in the thick of the storm.

When I look back to the time before my road ended, I realize that I regularly practiced enduring hardship in various arenas of my life: I trained as a runner, I stretched myself through educational opportunities, I practiced spiritual disciplines, and I said no to unhealthy eating. All of this taught my mind to run my body. General George Patton advised, "Make the mind run the body. Never let the body tell the mind what to do. The body will always give up."

The model of Nelson Mandela

Nelson Mandela inspired millions by his example of courage, tenacity, and transformational leadership. He remained strong and endured incredible adversity partially due to his commitment to preparation. Because he was deeply committed to the development of his mind, body, and spirit, he was well prepared for what came his way. Mandela said, "It is what we make out of what we have, not what we are given, that separates one person from another."

Mandela was a strong believer in education, both formal and informal. He wrote, "Education is the great engine of personal development. It is through education that the daughter of a peasant can become a doctor, that the son of a mine worker can become the head of the mine, that a child of farm workers can become the president of a great nation." [55] Even during his painful and challenging years in prison, Mandela fought for his own education and acted as a catalyst for the learning of others. He could have shrunk back and given up, but he didn't. He kept learning, read on a wide range of topics, initiated stimulating conversations with his prison mates and guards, and expressed his thoughts secretly through writing.

You can acquire an education that will prepare you for life in all sorts of places. You can learn in the classroom as well as from mentors, parents, coaches, advisors, counselors, friends, and other influential people. You can learn by reading, attending seminars and workshops, and listening to podcasts and webinars. I learned from all of them. You can learn in group discussions where you evaluate your own experience and the experience of others. You can learn through exposure to different cultures and experiences. You can learn from failure and success. Life is a learning laboratory filled with opportunities to prepare for life now and in the future.

Four approaches to learning that strengthen preparation

According to James M. Kouzes and Barry Z. Posner, there are four approaches to learning that tie directly into the way we prepare ourselves for life's challenges. The first approach is to learn by taking action. Those who learn this way jump in first and learn by trial and error. The second approach is to learn by thinking. Those who learn this way learn by reading articles, books, and online resources. The third approach is to learn by feeling. Those who learn this way confront themselves and ask themselves what they are worrying about. The fourth approach is to learn by accessing others. Those who take this approach learn by bouncing their hopes and fears off people they trust.[56]

Not everyone prepares or learns the same way. I have used all four approaches in my preparation. By taking a broad and holistic approach, I was able to move the learning from my head to my heart to my hands and feet. I learned the truth of Stephen R. Covey's advice: "To know and not to do is really not to know. To learn and not to do is not to learn."

Three practical steps to prepare for what's ahead

Two species of birds live in the desert. One bird wakes up in the morning, and all it can think about is, "Where is some dead meat?" The other bird wakes up, and all it can think about is, "Where are those colorful, sweet-smelling flowers where I can find some tasty nectar?" Each bird (the vulture and the hummingbird) finds exactly what it goes looking for. What it prepares to go after is exactly what it finds. The vulture finds what was alive in the past but is dead and rotting today. The hummingbird finds what is alive in the present, promising life and sweetness.[57]

Every day, we choose to be like the vulture or the hummingbird. We focus on bad news and negativity, or we go looking for opportunities to serve, bringing good to others and radiating optimism and hope.

During the re-entry phase, I realized how important it was to go out and find what was sweet and alive every day. I wanted to have an impact on people, regardless of where I was in the re-entry process. I wanted to find ways to encourage and help people — and make the world a better place. To do that, I took three practical steps every day that helped me prepare for what was coming.

1. I woke up and nurtured a positive mindset.

Every morning, I chose to cultivate a growth mindset. I took time to input positive thoughts and words into my mind. I journaled, prayed, reflected, and planned before starting my work. When worry was weighing me down, I worked hard to turn it over to God. When limiting beliefs were paralyzing me from action, I learned to reframe those beliefs to provide solid ground on which I could build.

2. I walked towards daily activities with a sense of purpose.

Frequently, I reminded myself why I did what I did. It wasn't enough for me to keep busy — I needed to spend time preparing myself for "purposeful" action, not just busy work. I needed to practice living on purpose every day because that is where life is found. At times, I had to regroup and take two steps back after taking three steps ahead, but purpose kept me going.

3. I ended each day celebrating and rehearsing the good.

The end of the day presents an opportunity to stoke the fire of optimism and delight. I made it my intention to avoid letting bad news fill my mind as the last thing before going to bed. Awareness of the world is one thing; being negatively impacted and dragged down is quite another. I learned to rehearse and count my blessings before going to sleep each night. This also was great preparation for doing it all over again the next day.

Detour Reflections

❖ On a scale of 1-10 (1 being totally unprepared and 10 being well prepared), what number do you give yourself on storm preparedness?

❖ What habit needs to be developed so you are better prepared for adversity?

Chapter 22: Work

"What purpose and place does work serve in my life?" That was one key question I asked myself when I was making my transition back into the real world of work after the detour. As I imagined the kind of worker I wanted to be, I came across a story of a boy who inspired me. The boy, leaning against the wall of a barber shop, dialed his phone and began speaking to the lady on the other end. The barber listened in.

Boy: Ma'am, I'm wondering if you would hire me to cut your lawn? (Pause) But I'll cut it for half the price of the person who cuts it now. (Pause) But, ma'am, I'll even sweep your sidewalk, so on Sunday you will have the prettiest lawn in all of Palm Beach! (A moment later, he hung up.)

Barber: I couldn't help but overhear…Did you get the job?

Boy: No.

Barber: Well, I like your attitude, and I'd like to offer you a job.

Boy: No, thanks.

Barber: But you were begging for a job on the phone just now, weren't you?

Boy: No, sir, I was just checking my performance at the job I already have. I am the one who currently cuts that lady's lawn.

There are several qualities I see and want to emulate in this story. The boy had a desire to do his work to the best of his ability. He had the courage to find out how he was *really* doing. He loved going the second mile when helping others. He was creative and resourceful. He appreciated feedback and found a way to get it. He was not afraid to hear the truth so he could keep improving.

What I learned about work during recovery

Since I wasn't able to work in an official capacity during my recovery, I needed to find a definition of work broad enough to include the work I was actually doing but not getting paid to do. I needed a definition that fit my reality. I actually found it in the dictionary. Work is: "activity involving mental or physical effort done in order to achieve a purpose or result."[58]

That definition didn't say I had to have a *job* to be doing *work*. It said that if I was engaged in activities involving mental and physical effort that achieved a purpose or result, I was working. Like the boy outside the barber shop, I saw in a whole new way what really mattered—*how* I did *what* I did mattered, regardless of whether it was official work or not. It mattered how I exercised my leg back into usability at the physiotherapy clinic, stayed out of the way of the house cleaner, volunteered at church, visited health care professionals, connected with neighbors, and helped a friend on his journey. If I did these activities on purpose and in a way that mattered, I knew I had made a positive impact and could fit it into a higher purpose.

How I answered certain questions also mattered. Did I give my best to what I was doing? Did I welcome feedback so I could keep improving? Did I go the second mile in the activities I was doing? Did I keep looking for ways to keep growing? I regularly asked my physiotherapist, "Is there anything else I should be doing to keep improving?" The answer often came back: "No, just keep doing what you're doing." Sometimes, however, I would be given a new insight, perspective, or idea that kept me working.

Being busy is not enough

We have an epidemic of "busy." Maybe it is because of all the options we currently have—250,000 apps for the iPhone, 387 breakfast cereals, unlimited entertainment options, downsizing at work that has created more work for those who are left, over-

154

committed children, which leads to over-committed parents (or the other way around).

I bristle when I hear someone say with pride, "I'm so busy!" That someone used to be me. I used to equate busy with "I'm important," "I'm productive," and "I feel alive." I have since changed my view. Part of that change occurred when work was stripped away from me and I was left to figure out what to do with my time while I recovered. What I came to realize was that it wasn't good enough to simply find things to do. I needed to find meaningful things to do. Being busy without a point left me tired and empty. Being busy on purpose left me satisfied and fulfilled. It was good to be busy, but only if I was contributing to others and serving the greater good.

Finding purpose in work

Work (paid or unpaid) is only meaningful if it has a purpose. It wasn't necessarily easy, but I did eventually find meaningful things to do—after a process of reflection, dialogue, and trial and error. That discovery process was aided by two exercises I found helpful.

The first exercise was to imagine a huge billboard on the edge of town. On that billboard, I was given the freedom to write or draw any message I liked. Thousands of people would pass by every day and look at the sign. I asked myself: What message should I put on the billboard? What would impact everyone who read it?

The second exercise was to imagine myself at a ripe old age sitting on a porch in a rocking chair with close friends and family nearby. As we sat there, everyone would start telling stories and speaking of the difference I had made in their lives. What would I want them to say?

The purpose that kept me anchored throughout my recovery was phrased something like this: "I am a lighthouse who helps people find their way." This purpose did not depend on having full mobility or being employed in a full-time job. I realized that there were activities I could participate in that would allow me to help and encourage people who needed some guidance and support for their journey. I discovered how meaningful "busy on purpose" can be. My "work" included the following activities and attitudes:

- **Put people first.**

If your "busy" hurts or neglects people, it's off base. Einstein said, "Only a life lived for others is worth living."

- **Learn from failure.**

You are going to make mistakes and over-commit from time to time. The key is to stop beating yourself up. Learn from your mistakes and commit to doing better next time.

- **Keep moving forward.**

Persistence is critical in purposeful living. It's not how well you start but how well you finish that really matters. Never give up working towards a life lived on purpose. Goethe said, "The greatest thing in this world is not so much where we stand, as in what direction we are moving."

- **Include God in your purpose.**

My conviction is that a life purpose without God will ultimately fail. I believe that God helped me find meaningful work during my recovery, which enabled me to avoid the despair that has come to many in similar situations.

Pushed or pulled

As I started the process of integrating my recovery journey with my emerging new normal, I received some help from my therapist. He asked me a question that struck at the heart of my relationship with work. He asked me, "Are you *pushed* by a drivenness to work and get things done or are you *pulled* by a desire to live from a place of value and deeper meaning?" As I pondered his question, I realized how I have often been more pushed than pulled. I get things done because I push through on projects, but that can create problems. I almost burned out once due to the pressure I put on myself to reach certain unreasonable expectations. I look back with gratitude on the people who guided me away from the burnout cliff that would have led to brokenness and exhaustion.

The danger signs I learned to recognize in my pre-accident life continued to be valuable tools while getting back onto the main road. These danger signs included unsettled anxiety, taking on too much, failing to take care of my body, neglecting my soul, lack of intellectual stimulation, and a shortage of quality time with friends. I realized that if certain things were lacking — reading good books, riding my scooter when the sun was shining, writing in my journal, taking time to connect with God and people — I was pushing, not pulling, my way forward. On the other hand, there were many benefits to being pulled along by deeper meaning:

- I felt at peace even with a long list of things to do.
- I took on tasks that aligned with my values and purpose.
- I was in a place where I knew when to adjust my activities to be more productive.
- I was able to deepen my learning.
- I had time to develop quality friendships.
- I ended up giving myself to others because I wanted to and not because I had to.

Final thought

When I realized work was any mental or physical activity done in order to achieve a greater purpose, I felt a deep satisfaction that was hard to explain. Ralph Waldo Emerson said: "The purpose of life is not to be happy. It is to be useful, to be honorable, to be compassionate, to have it make some difference that you have lived and lived well."

Detour Reflections

❖ What is your definition of work?

❖ What are you busy doing that you would describe as purposeful activity? If it is not purposeful, what needs to change to make it so?

157

Chapter 23: Change

There was an overarching theme I learned to embrace during recovery and re-entry into my new normal—the willingness to work with change. When do people change? John Maxwell says it is "when they *hurt* enough that they have to, *learn* enough that they want to, or *receive* enough that they are able to." During my recovery journey, all three were true.

In any change, there is something or someone who enters the picture and acts as the catalyst for change. My accident was the catalyst for a myriad of changes in my life. I was forced to change my shallow view of suffering. My previous view of work had left me empty-handed, and so that needed to change. My strong independent spirit had to change so that I would be willing to receive help. I changed because I was hurt and was compelled to change. I changed because I had learned enough that I was able to change. I changed because I received enough help to make it possible to change. In this chapter, I share various insights I picked up along the way that helped me change and grow.

Six principles to guide the change journey

What helped me navigate the messiness of change was to discover several key principles that could guide the change process. Change can be messy, but, thankfully, I was able to identify general patterns through study and observation. The disappointing news was that I discovered it was one thing to understand these principles and practices in my head and quite another to live them out in practice. This list isn't exhaustive, but it is a great place to start.

1. Change rarely happens instantaneously.

Deep change takes time. The sooner I accepted that, the better.

2. Change includes rewiring of the brain.

The reason change takes time is that new habits and thinking patterns take time to develop. You didn't get to where you are in your thinking overnight, and you won't rewire your brain overnight either.

3. Change is a process, not an event.

Change is a journey, not a destination. It is true that change can sometimes appear to happen quickly, like an event, but this overlooks the process that led to that point and the work that must still be done afterward. Real change takes time to take root.

4. Change includes certain steps, but the order may vary.

There is no perfect pattern that is true every time change happens, but there are steps that are usually present.

5. Change can be emotionally messy and involve grief and loss.

When you go through the change process, expect pain and emotion. It is normal.

6. In order for change to happen, you must embrace change.

Change doesn't happen just by thinking about it. It must be seized and embraced.

Six steps to take during the change journey

The change principles listed above form a foundation for change, but you then need to know the necessary steps to take to move through the change process. The following six steps, developed by Terry Bacon and Karen Spear,[59] helped me measure my progress as I walked my way through change.

1. Awareness

I began the change process when I became aware that change was needed. This awareness first came when I woke up from my drug-induced sleep and started wrestling with the reality of my broken body. I realized fairly quickly that getting better was going to require a willingness to adapt and change. That awareness resurfaced again and again, in response to different stimuli, telling me, "Change is coming. Get ready!"

2. Urgency

The cousin of awareness is urgency. Without urgency (defined as the recognition of "something important demanding swift action"), there isn't enough motivation to make the change. In the fall of 2011, I realized my recovery was going to require years, not months. That realization took me to a low point, smashed my expectations, and created a gigantic need for a major perspective change.

3. Deciding

With awareness and urgency pulling me forward, I was ready to make a decision to change. The decision to change gave me power to get moving and a firm place to go back to when I started to lose the motivation to keep going. The decision also included a willingness to ask for help since the emotional bottom I experienced was unlike any I had faced prior to this point. The decision to change opened the door for me to enter into psychotherapy.

4. Problem solving

It wasn't enough to make a decision to change. I needed to do the hard work of going down into my problems and dealing with them at a root level. I worked with others to solve the problems I faced, whether physical, spiritual, or emotional. Orthopedic surgeons and the rest of the medical community worked with me to solve the problems related to my broken and infected body. I cooperated with them, which aided in my recovery. Psychologists and other wise people worked with me to solve the problem of a broken and depressed spirit. Problem solving was a collaborative process, and it resulted in positive and lasting change.

5. Commitment

Once I started down the road to get the help I needed to change and heal emotionally, there were still days when I wanted to give up. Whenever giving up came to my mind, however, I thought about what I really wanted and about the commitment I had made to myself and others to get well. I couldn't control the outcome, but I could decide to move through the change process with courage.

Ken Blanchard said, "There's a difference between interest and commitment. When you are interested in doing something, you do it only when it is convenient. When you are committed to something, you accept no excuses."

6. Reinforcement

When I started into the change process with the therapist, I didn't know how long it would take. Could I experience the healing I wanted in one or two months? It ended up taking fourteen months. Change wasn't quick or easy, and it required the reinforcement of new support structures and new patterns of behavior. Because the recovery detour was messy, I needed ongoing reinforcement emotionally, spiritually, relationally, and physically.

Change involves risk

In order to change my thinking, my character, my behavior, and my body, I had to travel to places I had never been before. I had to risk appearing weak and foolish. I had to try things more than once because on the first attempt I would fail. This poem inspired me to risk and stick to the change journey when I was tempted to quit:

> To laugh is to risk appearing a fool,
> To weep is to risk appearing sentimental.
> To reach out to another is to risk involvement,
> To expose feelings is to risk exposing your true self.
> To place your ideas and dreams before a crowd is to risk their loss.
> To love is to risk not being loved in return,

To hope is to risk despair,

To try is to risk failure.

But risks must be taken because the greatest hazard in life is to risk nothing.

The person who risks nothing, does nothing, has nothing, is nothing.

He may avoid suffering and sorrow,

But he cannot learn, feel, change, grow or live.

Chained by his servitude he is a slave who has forfeited all freedom.

Only a person who risks is free.[60]

Risk is defined as "acting in spite of the possibility of injury or loss." To risk is to be alive, and to be alive requires change. Risk avoiders always play it safe and make every decision based on the possible dangers associated with that decision. Risk avoiders try to dance without moving their feet and to live without making any changes.

There is risk in doing physical things such as riding motorcycles and jumping out of airplanes. There is also risk when we love, laugh, weep, reach out, expose feelings, try, hope, and place our ideas out there for all to read. The choice I made with Vicky was to not buy another motorcycle, largely because of the risk. What I did not choose was to eliminate risk from my life. To do that would be to remove growth, discovery, and change. With risk comes the possibility of hurt but also the possibility of positive change.

Three ways risk changed me for the better

1. Risk allowed me to learn new skills and make new friends.

During my recovery, I sharpened my writing skills and took the risk of overcoming my insecurities about writing. I saw myself being able to help people with my words. I learned how to self-publish, resulting in a book (*Between Pastors*) that has impacted hundreds of people. I took the risk to set stretch goals and take action steps to achieve those goals. I became friends with total strangers and risked being vulnerable, which resulted in lasting connections and an enlarged supportive community.

2. Risk took me in a new direction and made me feel alive.

As soon as I could bend my knee 120 degrees, I bought a full-suspension mountain bike. It was way more bike than I needed at the time, but I bought it because I wanted to grow into this new sport. The first time I went for a ride down a real mountain bike trail with my mountain bike mentor, I was scared to death. I thought, "What am I doing?" But, as I continued to ride and risk falling, I felt a growing sense of aliveness.

3. Risk introduced me to new ways to increase my impact.

At one point in my recovery, I wanted to participate in a leadership training event. There was only one problem—I couldn't get to the event due to my immobility, and I had limited stamina for being out in public. I decided instead to create some DVDs and do the training that way. I had never done this before, but I said, "Why not?" I had a colleague record the sessions, and I edited the recordings to produce the DVDs. I learned a new skill and impacted others at the same time.

Motivation and the 5 + 1 influencers for change

When it comes to lasting change, no one can really motivate you except you—not your mother, your spouse, your doctor, your boss, your coach, or your therapist. According to Terry Bacon and Karen Spear,[61] people are more likely to be motivated to change when the following 5 + 1 influencers are present:

1. Fear

If people fear the consequences of things not changing, urgency for change increases. One of my motivators was the fear of losing the skills I'd developed prior to the accident. I knew that if I didn't practice my coaching skills, I'd lose my effectiveness as a coach. Therefore, the fear of losing the skill motivated me to find people I could coach for free just to stay sharp.

2. Fulfillment

The human need to climb to a higher level of achievement or accomplishment can be a strong influencer for change. I caught a glimpse of what it would be like to be a published author. I did not know everything that would be required, but, by working hard and learning new skills, I got my first book published.

3. Fellowship

People will change because they have a strong need to be part of a community where they find acceptance and belonging. I felt positive peer pressure and acceptance from my friends and family during my recovery, and this motivated me to keep growing and changing even when I would have been tempted to coast. I didn't want to let them down.

4. Followership

Change can come from the inspiration received from a leader. We must buy into the vision and decide to be part of it, but when we do, it can give us a greater sense of meaning and ignite our passion. A story I read early on in my recovery was the remarkable recovery journey of Matt Long.[62] He endured much worse than I did and inspired me to change and grow throughout my recovery.

5. Faith

Some people are influenced to change because they come to believe in something or someone greater than themselves. A pivotal part of my recovery was my personal belief in God. I daily surrendered to his leadership and to the work he wanted to do in my life. Words are inadequate to describe how my faith in God motivated me to keep trusting and looking past what I had lost to see what I had left.

+1 A traumatic event

One last motivator for change is the X factor of a traumatic event. This fits my story perfectly. The traumatic event I experienced had multiple layers and served as a catalyst for change. The radical nature of the recovery process propelled me to look for different ways to live and grow. The pain and shock changed my perspective and resulted in new directions, new behaviors, and significant change.

Detour Reflections

❖ What risk do you need to take today that will result in positive change and growth?

❖ Which of the 5 +1 influencers for change needs your attention to increase the potential for successful change in your life?

Chapter 24: Mindset

One of the supporting structures needed when rebuilding your life after a major setback is a proper mindset. The right mindset during the detour and re-entry won't change your circumstances, but it will give you inner strength *in* your circumstances.

Zig Ziglar said, "You are what you are and where you are because of what has gone into your mind. You can change what you are and where you are by changing what goes into your mind." As I made my way back to my new normal, the battle in my mind was fierce. I had changed. My circumstances had changed. The world around me had changed. Therefore, being able to maintain the right mindset was critical. I discovered that there are two basic mindsets[63] to choose from and making the right choice would be crucial.

Two basic mindsets

The first mindset is a fixed mindset. It is the belief that you have a limited amount of intelligence, personality, and character at your disposal and that these amounts are fixed and permanent.

The second mindset is a growth mindset. A growth mindset is the belief that your qualities and talents can be developed and increased through effort. Therefore, what determines your potential success is the amount of drive, energy, and determination you put into your task or goal.

When I learned of the distinction between the two, I jumped all over the growth mindset. I evaluated my work, play, and relationships with the view that I had the potential to expand and grow far beyond where I'd been before. I realized that I could let my new physical limitations limit me or build on the abilities I had left to expand what I could accomplish.

An example from history

The familiar Bible story of David and Goliath[64] is a perfect example of the two mindsets. The people of Israel, under the leadership of King Saul, were bogged down in their fight against the Philistines. Goliath stood in their way. He was almost ten feet tall, wore 126 pounds of armor, and put a paralyzing fear within every Israelite soldier. King Saul's army had a fixed mindset. The soldiers were convinced they didn't have the talent or ability to win. They believed they had reached the limit of their resources and could go no further.

Then David walked into the camp. David was a shepherd boy who was bringing lunch to his older brothers. When he heard Goliath taunting the Israelites and making fun of their God, he responded with a growth mindset. He quickly volunteered to fight the giant when he saw no one else stepping up to meet the challenge. David wasn't limited by a fixed mindset. Instead, he believed that, with God's help and his prior experience of killing lions, he could defeat the giant. Empowered by his growth mindset, David killed Goliath.

An example from education

It is a common belief that praise is necessary to instill confidence and inspire achievement in students. But the kind of praise and the mindset that is developed as a result of that praise makes a noticeable difference.

A study was conducted with two groups of adolescent students.[65] One group received praise for their ability and special talent. The other group were praised for their hard work and effort. Both groups were equal in IQ initially, but over time the students who received praise for their natural talent and intelligence saw their test scores drop. They felt inadequate, had high anxiety, felt the need to constantly prove themselves, and eventually gave up. The other group, who had been told they were hard workers, developed a growth mindset and welcomed harder and harder tests because they believed that if they worked harder, they could improve and succeed—and they did.

It is not intelligence or raw talent that determines success in life but our mindset. If we believe in our ability to grow, learn, and adapt to a changing situation, we will expand our capacities beyond what we thought was possible. However, if we believe our best days are behind us and we have reached the limit of our potential, our fixed mindset will cause us to settle and shrink back.

My best days were ahead of me

As I started to focus on re-entry into the ordinary world of regular work after more than three years spent in recovery, my greatest asset was not my raw talent or ability. My greatest asset was the belief that hard work, effort, and continuous learning would take me to where I needed to go. As I learned to let go of my past and the opportunities I had had previously, I found room to expand and grow into who I needed to become. A growth mindset gave me courage to wake up each day, learn what I needed to learn, and adapt to the new conditions I was living with. If I had rested on my past achievements or tried to recreate what I had lost, I would have missed out on the new possibilities that lay ahead.

A "grab and go" attitude

When a kitten gets into trouble, its mother comes and gently picks it up by the neck, taking it to safety. A baby monkey, on the other hand, must grab onto the back of its mother if it wants to make an escape. One is rescued, and the other rescues itself.[66] The kitten is limited by a fixed mindset, while the monkey has embraced the power of a growth mindset.

When I found myself in trouble, I was tempted to let others rescue me, but then it dawned on me: "If I sit here and wait to be rescued, opportunity will pass me by."

How do we get from where we are to where we want to go? How do we find the right opportunities, meet the right people, learn the right skills, shake off the bad habits, and chase after our dream? We embrace a growth mindset and grab hold of the opportunities that stand before us.

Like the monkey, when I was in trouble, I jumped onto opportunity's back. I learned new skills, met new people, took new risks, and prepared myself for the work I wanted to be doing. Seth Godin says, "No one is going to pick you. Pick yourself." I decided that instead of waiting for someone to help me, I was going to pick myself to be the person who would add value and provide help to those waiting for me to find them.

Balancing limits with a growth mindset

One of the challenges of adopting a growth mindset is learning how to deal with limitations. Limitations, whether real or imaginary, can paralyze us from moving forward. But not all pronouncements of limitations are negative. Some limits are presented as a reality check we desperately need.

Very early in my recovery, a physiotherapist told me I'd never run again. I did not receive her words well. In fact, I rejected them outright. I left the exercise room angry and vowed to prove her wrong. When I heard the same prognosis several months later, after several reconstruction surgeries on my leg, I was more open to the news. Eventually, I accepted my limitations and focused on what I had to work with. I used a growth mindset to see new possibilities while at the same time accepting my limitations. It helped that the physiotherapist delivering the news the second time was a person whom I trusted, who had experience I valued, and who spoke with compassion. Eventually, my new reality intersected with my optimism.

Five lessons that helped me reconcile limits with a growth mindset

1. Knowing your limits is the beginning of wisdom.

If you live with no awareness of your limits, you'll end up trying to do what you always did — and fail miserably. When things happen to us, we must adjust. If I had stayed angry with the first physiotherapist, I would only have hurt myself and limited my potential for growth. My physical condition was radically different, and I needed to accept the change in order to grow forward. Even Clint Eastwood said, "Men must know their limitations."

2. Having limits to overcome makes life exciting.

You can look at your limits and get depressed, or you can look at your limits and see an exciting challenge to overcome. I chose the latter. I chose to do the type of exercise I could do and not fixate on what I used to be able to do. When I rediscovered cycling, I knew I had found an activity I could grow with.

Helen Keller said, "The marvelous richness of human experience would lose something of rewarding joy if there were no limitations to overcome. The hilltop hour would not be half so wonderful if there were no dark valleys to traverse."

3. Adjusting to your new normal is possible.

Because I was willing to grow internally, I was able to change on the outside as well. If I had stayed fixated on "I have to run to be happy," I would have been miserable and stuck. Instead, I related to Helen Keller, who said, "I seldom think about my limitations, and they never make me sad. Perhaps there is just a touch of yearning at times; but it is vague, like a breeze among flowers."

4. You will get a higher return by focusing on what's left, not on what's lost.

I cannot count the number of times I've repeated the mantra, "Focus on what's left, not on what's lost." Focusing on what's left

171

created an expectation for new possibilities to emerge. T.F. Hodge said, "In the game of life, we all receive a set of variables and limitations in the field of play. We can either focus on the lack thereof or empower ourselves to create better realities with the pieces we play the game with."

5. It's an adventure to discover new ways to stay physically fit.

Instead of looking at running as my only option, I explored other options. In my search for options, I quickly thought of cycling, which had been a favorite pastime growing up. I live next door to some of the best mountain biking terrain in the country, and I have friends who mountain bike. I discovered the world of mountain biking was next for me.

Final thought

When I asked my physiotherapist what the chances were that I would be able to cycle, his reply was, "You have a 100 percent chance of doing that!" Those were odds I could live with. Brandon A. Trean said, "Stopping at limits is for those who lack a well-harnessed imagination."

Detour Reflections

❖ How would you describe your mindset? What is the result of that mindset?

❖ What are some practical ways to balance your limits with a growth mindset?

Chapter 25: Rhythm

Old Fred had lived a good life and was now lying in a hospital bed near the end of his life. The family was gathered around, along with their pastor, who had come to say a few words and offer some encouragement. As the pastor stood next to the bed, old Fred's condition appeared to deteriorate, and he motioned frantically for something to write on. The pastor lovingly handed him a pen and a piece of paper. Old Fred used his last bit of energy to scribble a note and then died.

The pastor, out of respect, thought it wise not to look at the note right then, so he placed it in his jacket pocket to read later. At the funeral, he was nearing the end of his message when he realized he was wearing the same jacket he had had on when old Fred handed him the note. He pulled it out and said, "You know, Fred handed me a note just before he died. I haven't looked at it, but, knowing Fred, I'm sure there's a word of inspiration and encouragement here for all of us." He opened the note and read out old Fred's last words: "Please step to your left. You're standing on my oxygen tube!"

Finding rhythm

Just like old Fred, who was robbed of life because he couldn't get oxygen, we are robbed of life if the things we need are cut off. Two things that can rob us of life are over-work (over-commitment) and excessive rest (too much leisure). I am familiar with both.

When the road ended, I was forced to rest and recover. Work stopped, and the pace of life slowed to a crawl. The rhythm during recovery went something like this: Eat. Sleep. Stretch. Nap. Operate. Medicate. Recover. Sleep. Read. Eat. Visit. Nap. I adjusted to that rhythm and had enough air to function with purpose and meaning. Eventually, however, as I moved into the re-entry phase,

I needed to add some work back into the equation. I started slowly at first but eventually filled my time with meaningful "work-like" activities. These activities included writing, reading (to learn something practical or useful), helping people, coaching (on a volunteer basis), and advising/counseling people in need. I still took the necessary time to rest, heal, and recover, but, as time went on, I contributed more and more.

The farther I traveled down recovery road, the closer I got to a new normal and the more important it was to find balance between work and rest. I discovered five principles that guided me back to balance and rhythm.

1. Identify the signs that work or rest is too dominant.

Rhythm is like a piece of classical music written for a symphony. It has notes that are played by various instruments but also rests that create important gaps between the notes. Work without rest increases stress, saps vitality, and produces discord. I studied my patterns of rest and work to find the music I needed to play.

2. Describe your life as you would like it to be and why that is important.

Something happens when you write down your intentions and the reason why those intentions are important. I kept a journal where I wrote my thoughts and feelings as well as my hopes and dreams. Writing out my future desires changed my expectations and influenced my daily activities. Having a why helped me find my way.

3. Find work you enjoy and are good at.

Rest alone is not enough. We need to complement our rest with work that brings enjoyment and that we can do well. We were created to do just that. Rabbi Lapin said, "Don't follow your passion. Find work that serves people, and learn to love your work."

4. Find healthy activities that give you rest.

Not everything that looks restful replenishes the body, mind, and spirit. What I looked for was ways to rest at the core of who I was. One activity that provided that was bike riding. Yes, it was exercise, but it also replenished my mind and soul. Getting eight hours of sleep after offloading my stress and anxiety provided true rest. A nap in the middle of the day did something similar.

5. Enlist friends and partners to support you in finding rhythm.

I am much more interdependent than I used to be. I have learned to see the important role other people have to play in my life. I need them to speak into my life and help me stay in rhythm.

A lesson from Ethan Edwards

In the movie *The Searchers*, Ethan Edwards, played by John Wayne, joins up with a few ranchers to chase down some Indians who have stolen their cattle. After they have ridden out into the desert, they realize it's a trap to lure them away from their ranches and they must turn around and go back. At this point, Ethan says, "No, if we head right back, we'll kill the horses. We need to rest and feed the horses before we go back." The other ranchers disagree and start riding back. Sure enough, after Ethan has fed and rested his horses and started on his return journey, he comes across the other ranchers—who are on foot because their horses have all died.

Rhythm breathes life into your whole being.

Take the next step

More than once, I felt overwhelmed as I tried to claw my way back and find a healthy rhythm between work and rest. At times, the harder I tried, the harder it seemed to get. I was distracted by interruptions and had difficulty keeping motivated and focused. The problem was that I would feel overwhelmed by whatever task

I was facing and would freeze into inactivity. Then I would find myself resting when it wasn't rest I needed but activity.

How did I cope with this challenge? I focused on the next step I needed to take. A wise author who inspired me as I worked my way back into regular work and a healthy rhythm was Henry Cloud.[67] His advice was simply: "If you want to achieve your goal, don't focus on how far you have to go. Focus on the next step of getting there. Just the next activity."

By the time I arrived at the three-and-a-half-year point of my recovery, I had experienced multiple stops and starts, numerous ups and downs. Finally, however, I was nearing the end of my recovery journey. I was feeling both hopeful and overwhelmed — hopeful because I could start to realize my new normal, but overwhelmed because there were so many steps I needed to take to get there.

Five key elements for next step living

Desire alone did not give me what I needed to reach my goals. Wanting to have a full coaching practice left me miles away from having it. I realized that I would have to work diligently for a long time in order to achieve my goals. My pendulum had been stuck in the resting position for so long that switching to an active, working lifestyle was going to take considerable effort. Henry Cloud taught me: "An idea without action is only a fantasy. A true dream, or vision, requires legs. Put a foot on the floor and get walking towards your vision."

The key ideas that nurtured next step living included:

1. Set clear learning goals.

The gap between where I was and where I wanted to be was not called "failure" but "learning." Learning offered me practical steps to get me where I hoped to be. Instead of being overwhelmed by what I didn't know, I chose to focus on what I needed to develop (skills, attitudes, competencies) so I could move forward towards my desired destination.

2. Practice solitude, but avoid isolation.

Henry Cloud advised: "We need solitude. But isolation is a cancer to the soul. Get enough proactive solitude and avoid defensive isolation. They are different." I learned to be comfortable with long periods of alone time while recovering. As work picked up, however, I learned to be conscious of when solitude had started to turn into isolation.

3. Learn to let pain travel with you.

Henry Cloud taught: "A surgeon doesn't suddenly yell, 'Oh, crap! He's bleeding!' He knows it's part of getting to a good outcome. Don't let a little pain scare you!" There is pain that helps and pain that hurts. The kind of pain I learned to embrace was the pain that made me stronger. Finding a healthy rhythm involved taking action, even if it was uncomfortable, because I knew the action would enable me to get to my destination.

4. Realize fear won't kill you.

Fear at times kept me from doing the activities I needed to do in order to move forward. Fear is often False Evidence Appearing Real. I learned to name my fear for what it was, recognize how false beliefs were limiting me, and step into a more empowering reality. Henry Cloud advised, "Try one new thing tomorrow that you have been wanting to do, but have been too afraid to do. Notice the fear did not kill you and then see what you learn."

5. Cut your work into bite-size pieces.

Henry Cloud taught: "Research proves the brain can't multitask. If you are doing something important, turn everything else off. It'll increase performance by 50 percent." It is hard to turn everything else off and focus on one thing at a time. Yet, finding rhythm and being productive demand it. I use the timer on my cell phone to focus on one thing at a time. I also find a location that is free from distraction and disturbance. Multitasking is not a friend of finding rhythm.

Detour Reflections

❖ How would you describe the state of your rhythm?

❖ What does it mean for you to focus on "the next step of getting there"?

Chapter 26: Resistance

There is a battle that rages whenever we try to do something great—something significant, something that will move us forward, something beyond what seems possible, something noteworthy. When the goal is progress, the battle we face will be with resistance.

When the road ended, resistance was everywhere, calling me to settle, to give up, to back down, to stay the victim, and to stop working hard. During the detour, resistance raised its ugly head every time I attempted to wake up my dormant and atrophied muscles. As I made my way back onto the road, resistance whispered, "Your best days are behind you," "You've become incompetent," and "You've lost your edge."

What activities are most commonly met with resistance? Steven Pressfield, in his book *The War of Art*, lists the following:[68]

- the pursuit of any calling in life, any creative art
- any diet or health regimen
- any program of spiritual advancement
- any program designed to overcome a bad habit or addiction
- education of any kind
- any act of moral or ethical courage
- any undertaking aimed at helping others
- any act that entails commitment of the heart
- the taking of any principled stand in the face of adversity

Pressfield says resistance will oppose "any act that rejects immediate gratification in favor of long-term growth, health, or integrity. Or, expressed another way, any act that derives from our higher nature instead of our lower."[69]

My goal as I made my way back into the mainstream of life was to integrate my new normal with regular life. The goal of resistance was to get me sidetracked from that goal into pursuing a much lesser one.

The many faces of resistance

Resistance is multi-faceted. Resistance is also invisible. We can't see it, but we can feel its negative pull. It tries to shove us away, distract us, prevent us from doing our best work. Resistance is internal and doesn't come from those around us (our spouse, our job, our circumstances, our physical condition). It is self-generated and self-perpetuated. Resistance is insidious. It will tell us anything to keep us from doing our work. It has no conscience, will double-cross us with deals, and is always lying. Resistance is also universal. I had to tell myself I was not the only one struggling with resistance. It affects everyone in some way.

Resistance never sleeps. The battle against resistance must be fought anew every single day, and it will even show up in the middle of the night. Resistance is fueled by fear but has no strength of its own. Every ounce of its energy comes from us. If we master our fear, we will conquer resistance. Whether it was getting back into shape physically, taking steps in order to get back to work, or completing a project I was working on, I had to choose to meet resistance head on. I resolved that resistance was not going to stop me in my tracks.

Ten handles and one key to dealing with resistance

I grabbed hold of certain handles that made it possible to deal with resistance without being overcome by it:

1. Show up every single day.
2. Work hard all day long.
3. Focus on what you can control
4. Keep your purpose in sight at all times.

5. Let go of what you can't control.

6. Pray and express gratitude on a daily basis.

7. Learn to live with less than ideal circumstances.

8. Stay committed for the long haul.

9. Get better at what you are doing and at who you are.

10. Take time to laugh and play a little every day.

In addition to these handles, there was a key distinction I needed to understand: there is a big difference between talking to yourself and listening to yourself. It is the difference between anxiety and confusion on the one hand and perspective and traction on the other. You are not crazy if you talk to yourself. Quite the contrary. It is a practice that is extremely helpful when dealing with resistance.

Maybe, like me, you have heard the voice that says, "You're probably going to fail. You'll never figure this out. Just give up and try something else. You're not qualified to do what you're attempting to pull off." Listening to yourself is a passive exercise that lets the negative tapes from your past play over and over again and dictate your attitudes and actions. Talking to yourself, on the other hand, is an active exercise. It helps you turn down the unproductive head noise, foster a positive attitude, and take productive action.

When I increased the time I spent working, I was met with resistance and plenty of head noise. The head noise created anxiety and was very challenging to deal with. I did not fight the resistance head on but diligently set reasonable goals and developed action plans to turn those goals into reality.

Once I started moving towards the completion of my goals, the noise created by resistance only got louder. It said, "You're not reaching your goals. What's wrong with you?" Then the accusations got even worse: "You don't have what it takes to do your job, do you? You've gotten soft because you've been off for so long."

As the noise continued, I called, "Time out!" I said to myself and anyone else who was listening (namely, resistance), "Something is off with this chatter going on inside my head." The voice made sense on one level, but on another level it felt like a bully. It was true that I wasn't reaching my goals as fast as I had hoped, but that didn't mean I wasn't making a difference or doing my job.

As the noise got louder, it was time to do some talking—to myself. I remember the day I had a heart-to-heart talk with myself while walking around the block. As I walked and pondered my reality, I realized I had set the bar way too high. I had expected a quicker return to full-time work. I also had been unrealistic about what another surgery would do to my momentum and productivity. I told myself that I needed to keep my expectations high enough to provide a push but not base my personal worth or value on achieving those expectations when doing so was outside my control. As I continued, I talked myself down from the anxious ledge of over-inflated expectations and perceived failure onto the firm ground of "You are making a difference. It's a season of sowing, not harvest, right now."

Principles to help you do less listening and more talking

- **Don't ignore what you are listening to.**

This may sound counterintuitive, but to try to ignore or suppress the inner chatter only increases its intensity and frequency. You don't have to agree with what you're hearing, but it's important to acknowledge the chatter and the feelings it creates.

- **Listen and learn from what you are hearing.**

The challenge in listening to your head noise is to hear what's being said but not allow the inner voice to bully you into worrying and having feelings of inadequacy. Being curious about what's being said can lead to new discoveries and help you separate truth from fiction.

- **Talk to yourself in order to stay active.**

The more you talk to yourself, the more power self-talk will have in your life. You can move into positive action by talking to yourself, reframing your situation, and speaking the truth. On one of my walks around the block, I had a breakthrough. I said to myself:

> You are having a bigger impact than you think. Having stretch goals hasn't been a bad thing because it has gotten you out of your comfort zone and opened up doors. You need to see the season you're in as a season of sowing, not harvest. Your season of launching out and harvest will come. Be ready for this next surgery when it comes. Do what you can until then. Keep adding value to the people you can help. You are taking action, doing important work. If you listen to this positive voice, you'll be a lot better off.

Telling say-so stories instead of so-so stories

Another approach that deals decisively with resistance is telling powerful future stories. A powerful future story pulls us forward through resistance. The positive future story we tell ourselves is our "say-so" story. I had a say-so story come true, and it was an experience I was able to build on. At 9:00 o'clock on a Saturday morning, a friend picked me and my mountain bike up in his truck and drove us to the parking area on Sumas Mountain. There is a park there with bike trails designed for riders of all levels, and people come from miles around to enjoy them. Long before this day came, I had had a say-so moment that cut through the resistance. The story I told myself three years before this first mountain bike ride was: "I will buy a mountain bike and learn to ride the local mountain trails." With fear and trepidation, I started down Squid

Line Trail on my first day of riding. What a powerful milestone moment that was!

What keeps people from telling themselves say-so stories?

- **fear** — "What if I fail and my say-so doesn't happen?"
- **apathy** — "I don't care if I grow and change."
- **anger** — "I hate my life! Life is so unfair."
- **self-pity** — "It's not up to me to get out of the mess I'm in."
- **bitterness** — "I will not forgive. I want to hold onto my injury and bitterness."
- **unbelief** — "I don't believe positive self-talk helps."

Habits that nurture a say-so life

1. Let your words paint a picture of your preferred future.

Say-so living is living in a future vision that is not yet realized but only seen in your imagination. Imagination helps break the chains of so-so thinking. Brandon Trean says, "Stopping at limits are for those who lack a well-harnessed imagination."

Solomon said, "Words kill, words give life; they're either poison or fruit — you choose"[70] and "The right word at the right time is like a custom-made piece of jewelry."[71]

2. Let limits inform your words but not define your dream.

There is a fine line between blind optimism and say-so living. Overcoming resistance is not about simply saying, "If I can dream it, I can achieve it." Say-so living is about having the strength, ability, talent, and resources to turn your future story into a reality.

When I started saying "I will mountain bike someday," I was on crutches and months away from walking. However, I had accepted the harsh reality that I would never run a marathon while also seeing the real possibility that I would eventually be able to ride a bike up and down a mountain.

3. Let your words shape your daily actions.

Predictions about the future are important, but they lack teeth if a daily plan to walk towards fulfilling those predictions isn't also in place. Say-so talk backed up by daily action is what will ultimately overcome resistance.

When I told myself my future mountain biking story, I had to support that dream with hours and hours of recumbent bike riding long before I was ready to ride a "real" bike. I had to keep struggling to do this while putting up with a knee that would only bend 85 degrees until another surgery increased my bend to 120 degrees.

Detour Reflections

❖ What voice seems loudest in your life?

❖ How can you do more talking and less listening?

Chapter 27: Momentum

When you have momentum, it is your friend. When you have lost momentum, you desperately want it back again. What is momentum? It is "the strength or force that something has when it is moving." It is also "the strength or force that allows something to continue or to grow stronger or faster as time passes."[72]

What causes momentum to be lost? Several factors, including life-altering events such as accidents, sickness, job loss, family tragedies, hurricanes, and tornadoes. Momentum can be lost as a result of inactivity that persists for too long or as a result of internal beliefs that grind progress to a halt.

When my road ended, I experienced a total loss of momentum. It was not just a blip on the momentum-o-meter. It was the most devastating loss of momentum I had ever experienced. Because the momentum lost was so great, the journey back was much more challenging than I had anticipated.

How to start regaining momentum

There were a few strategies I picked up as I clawed my way back from inactivity to active engagement and my eventual re-entry into regular life. These included the following:

1. Acknowledge you are stuck or stalled.

Regaining momentum starts with admitting you have lost it. There is something healthy about saying, "I have lost my momentum." When you admit you have lost something of value, you are more likely to be motivated to go looking for it. When I admitted I was stuck, it did not take away my motivation; rather, it clarified my reality and motivated me to plan a way forward.

2. Identify limiting beliefs.

The list of beliefs that can hinder the restoration of momentum is long. Some of mine were: "I'm afraid to try because I might fail. I'm not sure if I should go in this direction, so I had better wait until things are clearer. I'll wait until things are perfect before I start again. I shouldn't have to work to get momentum back again since it was stolen from me. There's got to be an easier way to regain the momentum I once had."

3. Assess your readiness to regain momentum.

It is unwise to assume you are ready to regain momentum if "brutal facts" say otherwise. At various stages of the detour, I desperately wanted to regain momentum in my fitness, work, and mobility, but the timing was just wrong. Eventually, however, I reached a point on the journey when I could get serious about getting fired up again.

4. Articulate clearly where you want to go.

A clear picture of what future momentum looks like is critical. The picture of the future you paint in your mind will spur you on when the going gets tough. I knew I could get serious about getting back to work after my surgeon told me that no more surgeries were needed on my right knee. That was a definite turning point in my ability to regain momentum. Immediately after that appointment, I set a goal to become an executive coach and signed up for a training program that would turn that intention into a reality.

5. Connect existing momentum to an area where you're stuck.

Momentum is contagious. If you want traction for growth and change in one area, tie that change to another area where you already have momentum. I had momentum in the area of writing since I had spent hundreds of hours in my recliner writing a book, blogging, and writing various articles. I also had momentum in the area of exercising and getting myself back into physical shape.

6. Connect with resourceful people.

There is a wise proverb that says, "None of us is as smart as all of us." Regaining lost momentum on your own is a steep hill to climb. It is much easier to regain lost momentum when you invite others to help. I invited friends, family, counselors, coaches, teachers, pastors, colleagues, and others to support me on the long road back. These resourceful people gave encouragement, perspective, advice, counsel, prayer, and support that made a noticeable impact.

The slinky affect

There is a lot to learn about momentum from the slinky. You regain lost momentum the same way you play with a slinky. Invented in 1945, this children's toy has given hours of pleasure to children all over the world. I received my first slinky as a boy and played with it for hours. I remember coaxing my slinky to start moving down the stairs until it eventually moved on its own. Once it started to move smoothly, I could step back and watch it do its magic. I was always amazed at how the shiny coiled spring moved effortlessly down the stairs without any help.

The slinky is a metaphor for the relationship between "what you do" and "the results you get." The initial coaxing of the slinky is like the discipline and hard work needed to get moving again. But once you gain momentum, much greater progress is achieved with much less work.

Applying the slinky effect to regain momentum wasn't some magic formula that brought instant results. Instead, it was a daily commitment to certain routines and practices that got me moving again. This involved coaxing myself physically, emotionally, spiritually, mentally, and professionally, one step at a time.

How exactly did I do it? In the area of physical fitness, this meant daily exercise, regular stretching, eating fewer yam fries, and physiotherapy, both at home and at the clinic. I also needed massive amounts of patience because I'd take three steps forward, then be forced to take two steps back. But I kept the bigger goal in mind, knowing that the better shape I was in when a setback happened, the quicker I would recover. My progress was slow but steady. When I first started riding the recumbent bike in my living room, it took me twelve minutes to go one kilometer. Eventually I got up to riding five kilometers in twenty-four minutes. When I was active, I lost weight, had more energy, reduced my stress, and increased my mobility.

In the area of emotional health, I coaxed the slinky down the stairs by monitoring my emotional gauges. When I saw I was in trouble, I took action to address the problem. When I felt depression settling down on me, I went back to the therapist to process what was troubling me. At other times, I went for coffee with empathetic, listening friends. I went for walks, journaled, and cried. I tried to match the emotional doldrums I was in with the right remedy.

In the area of mental and intellectual health, I coaxed the slinky down the stairs with reading, reflecting, journaling, listening to podcasts, and watching uplifting videos and TED (Technology, Entertainment, and Design) Talks. I planned my day's activities more consistently, initiated contact with people, prepared teaching materials, grew as a writer, learned how to self-publish, and never stopped expanding my mind.

In the area of spiritual health, I coaxed the slinky down the stairs by being aware of my soul's condition. I watched for signs of God's activity all around me, became more disciplined in reading the Bible and other spiritually uplifting material, and practiced prayer and meditation. I joined groups of like-minded people who wanted to grow and be supported in their spiritual journeys.

In the area of my professional life, I coaxed the slinky down the stairs by increasing the hours of work gradually but intentionally. I reintroduced routines and practices I knew would lead to work that satisfied and achieved results. I called potential clients, participated in networking activities, attended courses to improve my skills, met with key people, became more aware of opportunities to help people, set measurable work goals, hired outside professionals to work with me, and scheduled productive activities.

Regaining momentum is not a quick fix

Dave Ramsey said, "Discipline is not a microwave; it's a Crock-Pot." Regaining lost momentum takes time. At times, I waited months to see the results I imagined myself having. What I often didn't see was the growth that was taking place under the surface and which was, in fact, building the momentum that would become visible later on.

There are no shortcuts to rebuilding lost momentum. As with the slinky, success comes after careful coaxing and repeated effort, one step at a time. Each small success created just enough momentum to keep me pushing forward to the next step.

A final thought

To get your momentum back, Lorii Myers says you need a "big push." She says: "The BIG push means being able to develop and sustain momentum toward your goal; it is the process of actively replacing excuses with winning habits, the ultimate excuses blockers. Moreover, it is being willing to go to the wall for what you want or believe in, to push beyond your previous mental and physical limits, no matter what it takes."[73]

Detour Reflections

❖ Where are you stuck right now?

❖ What is a first step you could take to help you on your climb?

Chapter 28: Opportunity

Opportunity comes dressed in all kinds of disguises. It is often here one minute and gone the next. It usually demands a response sooner than later. In the words of Elyse Sommer, "Sometimes opportunity knocks like a loud windburst; more often it arrives like a burglar and disappears before you realize it was there."

Opportunity is defined as "an appropriate or favorable time or occasion" and "a situation or condition favorable for attainment of a goal."[74] Opportunity during the detour was a regular visitor. As I started to integrate my new normal with mainstream life, however, my senses were heightened as I looked for conditions favorable to the attainment of my goals and desires. The process of moving from seeing to seizing an opportunity took time and included the right mindset and the right approach.

Opportunity's attitude and mindset

- **Opportunity demands an attitude that says "yes" to risk.**

There is an imaginary line in the sand when it comes to risk and opportunity. You cross the line and decide to risk—perhaps because you have realized that staying where you are is actually the greater risk. There were times during the detour when I was limited in the risks I could take because my body wasn't ready. As I approached re-entry into normal life, however, the more I had to say "yes" to risk if I wanted to continue to grow.

- **Opportunity requires a willingness to take charge of our own growth and learning.**

When I embraced new experiences, watched for new insights, and opened myself up to new people, doors of opportunity opened up. Those doors led to growth in character, deeper friendships, the satisfaction received from helping others, and the opportunity to see my dreams come true. Instead of letting my down time get me down, I turned it into growth time. I signed up for on-line courses and challenged my mind to stretch and grow. I found a free university course on World Religions that I could take while sitting in my recliner. The writing courses I took gave me the tools to write on a daily basis, start a blog, and begin to help people with my words.

- **Opportunity requires us to turn "if only" into "if."**

"If only" is a phrase filled with regret and rear-view mirror living. It does not move us forward and keeps us from walking through the door of opportunity. "If only" is a fantasy.

Wishing for something to change in the past is a waste of energy. We need to grieve our losses and take time to heal from past hurts. But that process should get us ready to move forward, not keep us staring at past mistakes and misfortunes. The key to seizing opportunity is to drop "only" and keep "if." "If only" causes paralysis and keeps us focused on the past. "If" opens up creativity and options for the future.

Actions that turn the key in the door of opportunity

1. Just try.

I'd rather go through life saying, "At least I tried," than saying, "If only I had tried." Hockey player Wayne Gretzky said, "You miss 100 percent of the shots you don't take." Trying is all about getting up every day and using the talent, energy, and resources you currently have to make a difference. I look back on the months of my detour and can honestly say, "At least I tried." Not everything I tried worked, but my efforts opened many doors, and I found my life was worth living.

2. Go ahead and fail.

I learned to say, "That didn't work," instead of saying, "I can't do that because it might not work." Permission to fail is a gift you give yourself. Permission to fail helped release me from the paralysis of my insecurity and the fear of stepping out. A wise person once said, "I would rather live my life with mistakes made and lessons learned than to live it full of regrets, if only, and what could have been."

3. Just do something.

When I acted on the knowledge I had, it silenced the "if only" voice inside my head. When I did something productive and helpful for others, it took my mind off past regrets and disappointments. I found on many occasions that a change of scenery — talking to a stranger, listening to a hurting friend, writing a poem — changed my mood and my life. Someone else once said, "You can stand there thinking, 'if only,' or you can go, take charge, and change it."

4. Make some art.

I learned to stop saying, "If only I had some amazing talent such as the ability to paint a beautiful picture, I'd do something with my life!" Instead, I started saying, "Why don't I paint some word pictures and create some word art?" True art contains three elements: 1) it is made by a human being; 2) it is created to have an impact and to change someone else; and 3) it is a gift the artist offers to the world. If these three elements are present in your work or hobby or other endeavor, you are making art.[75]

5. Practice "nexting."

When I put the focus on what I would do next time, I stopped obsessing over how I failed last time. This is a technique called "nexting." For example, if you lock your keys in your car, instead of beating yourself up and calling yourself a loser, say to yourself, "Next time, when I get out of my car, I will reach into my pocket and make sure I can jingle my keys before I shut the door." Trust me – it works.

DETOUR

Opportunity is seized when you mine the gap

"Mining the gap" is an expression describing how we use the time between a disturbance and our response. If we react too quickly to something that happens to us, we may miss the opportunity to respond in a way that is more positive and productive. Mining the gap is all about pushing the pause button after a disturbing event in order to seize the opportunities that arise.

There is a powerful example of mining the gap in a story told by Viktor Frankl, a Jewish psychiatrist imprisoned in the death camps of Nazi Germany. He discovered the gap one day while sitting naked and alone in his small room. He became aware of his freedom to decide how his pain and suffering were going to affect him. Frankl wrote, "When we can no longer change a situation, we are challenged to change ourselves." He realized that between the stimulus (what had happened to him) and the response (how he would respond to what had happened to him) was the power to choose.[76] The gap may be very short in time, but when it is seized, it can make a powerful difference.

Mining the gap is about telling yourself a different story in the brief time between a stimulus and your response. In those few seconds, you must choose between slinging mud or digging for gold. Here are five practical ways to improve your gap mining skills:

1. Notice when your buttons are being pushed.

The place to begin is to notice when your buttons are being pushed. You can't fix what you can't see. As I started to notice button pushing, it made it possible for me to stop and think before reacting.

2. Pray the serenity prayer.

The Serenity Prayer was the food that my soul feasted on often. The words were especially helpful when I encountered the stimulus of suffering, confrontation, or conflict. I prayed, "God, grant me the serenity to accept the things I cannot change; courage to change the things I can; and wisdom to know the difference."

3. Tell an optimistic story.

You have two options when encountering harsh reality—either react negatively or find something positive to be grateful for or to do. As I made my way back into the mainstream of life, my leg complained often about how stiff it was. I didn't ignore what it was telling me. Instead, I embraced what I could do to help the situation, such as go for a bike ride, take a walk, or stand up and stretch. I focused on the story I wanted to tell—a story of perseverance, tenacity, and gratitude—not a story of trouble and complaining.

4. Remember what you value.

Remembering your values gives you a place to stand between stimulus and response. Whenever I needed to mine the gap and choose my next move carefully, I thought of the things that really mattered to me: my family, my faith, making a difference, being a life-long learner, and being real. Reflecting on my values enabled me to change the way I reacted.

5. Ask for feedback often.

None of us can see the whole picture, especially when we are under pressure from difficult events. I had numerous people speak into my life—friends, family members, colleagues, coaches, counselors, mentors, specialists, pastors, God, and even random people I met. I chose to be accountable to those who had my best interest in mind.

Detour Reflections

❖ What "if only" do you use?

❖ What action can you take today that will open the door to opportunity?

Chapter 29: Brokenness

The Japanese have an ancient craft known as *kintsugi*. It can be best understood this way: If a piece of valuable china is dropped and breaks, instead of throwing it away or repairing it perfectly, the *kintsugi* craftspeople use lacquer containing gold to piece it back together. The cracks in the china are celebrated and honored with golden seams. From that point forward, the restored bowl or vase is considered more beautiful than the original because of its healed brokenness.

The scars we carry in our lives, visible or invisible, give us the opportunity to tell a story of healed brokenness. When I look at my legs with their many scars, I see a shadow of my former self. I remember the days when I ran races, climbed hills, walked without a limp, and enjoyed perfect health. As I look at my beaten up-body, I face a daily choice. I can either mourn the loss of my once athletic legs and healthy body, or I can choose to embrace the new beauty found in the scars that are a permanent part of my new reality.

The pathway to healed brokenness

The pathway to healed brokenness is found in *kintsugi*. It is not enough to acknowledge our brokenness. We must also take the steps necessary to move towards healing, so brokenness can be transformed into beauty. Renewed hope comes as we pick up the pieces of our life and apply the appropriate glue and gold. The glue includes a new perspective, fresh courage, renewed purpose, divine strength, help from our friends, and the daily choice to let go of the past. Nicole Sobon observed, "Sometimes the hardest part isn't letting go but rather learning to start over."

I traveled this journey. I took my pain, brokenness, and limitations and offered them up as a gift to the world. I made a daily choice to not fixate on my scars nor to be embarrassed and ashamed of them. I learned to let my new reality be a testimony to the resilience I had discovered.

This journey of healed brokenness continues throughout life. Further events and experiences test and challenge us to keep accepting and surrendering our brokenness on a regular basis. I tried to practice the words of Harold J. Duarte-Bernhardt: "We are all broken and wounded in this world. Some choose to grow strong at the broken places."

The fruit of healed brokenness

Healed brokenness produced some noticeable fruit in my life. I developed empathy for those who suffer, a greater appreciation for life, patience during times of waiting, a stronger focus on inner beauty, a decreased focus on external perfection, and a heightened appreciation for the gifts and abilities I still had.

Next time you see someone walk with a limp, hear the story of a cancer survivor, talk to a new widow, listen to the struggle of someone living with mental illness, drive by a homeless man, or see the pain in the eyes of a mother who has lost her daughter to drugs, look deeper for signs of healed brokenness. If those signs aren't yet present, say a prayer that that person's life won't end with unhealed brokenness.

It is not easy to "turn our scars into beauty marks" It doesn't happen in an instant, but it is within the realm of what's possible.

A lesson from a shabby rabbit

Children's stories can speak to the child in all of us. *The Velveteen Rabbit* is the story of a child's toy who was deeply troubled by the arrival of fancier toys who acted superior to his simple and very worn self. Eventually, another toy, the Skin Horse, shared some wisdom that changed everything. He explained that it was possible for a toy to become "Real" if "a child loves you for a long, long time."

The Rabbit asked if becoming Real would hurt, and the Skin Horse replied, "When you are Real, you don't mind being hurt...Generally, by the time you are Real, most of your hair has been loved off, and your eyes drop out, and you get loose in the joints and very shabby. But these things don't matter at all, because once you are Real you can't be ugly, except to people who don't understand." One Christmas morning, the Rabbit finally became Real. The story concludes: The Rabbit "didn't mind how he looked to other people, because the nursery magic had made him Real, and when you are Real, shabbiness doesn't matter."[77]

Dealing with our own shabbiness

The events of life wear us down and create shabbiness we aren't always keen to embrace. This shows up as hair loss, memory loss, loss of beauty, loss of strength, disfigurement, and a general reduction of who we once were.

I'm not the strong, healthy person I used to be. My body has been marred by life-altering events. My legs don't work right, I walk with a limp, and I have scars that are impossible to hide in a swimming pool. It impacts how I see myself and how I show up in the world. I don't always feel "real" or alive when reflecting on my shabbiness.

Why is that? Is it because I sometimes let the voices around me impact how I feel about myself? Do I believe the lie that says, "You are real only if you are strong and put together"?

I learned two principles that helped me accept my shabbiness.

1. You can be real when you know you are loved.

The Rabbit knew he was loved and, because of that, was OK with his shabbiness. How about you? Do you know you are loved? Do you believe that God loves you? Do you love yourself, warts and all? Do you have someone in your life who loves you unconditionally? If you experience genuine love, you will have the capacity to accept your shabbiness and embrace the fact that you are real. I am so grateful to know that God loves me unconditionally. I'm also grateful to know that I'm loved by my family and friends, who have stood by me in all kinds of situations. That is a wonderful gift I never want to take for granted.

2. You can be real when you walk with humility.

Walking with humility involves two decisions. First, you must decide to be weak and vulnerable with others, to set aside your need to be perceived as strong. This means being comfortable in your own skin. I had to learn this, to learn to be myself — scars, limp, limitations, and all. The more you accept your own shabbiness and weakness, the more you can look honestly at yourself — and that may allow you to also see the character and worth that lie within your shabby exterior. Criss Jami said, "To share your weakness is to make yourself vulnerable; to make yourself vulnerable is to show your strength." The best gift you can give others is to be who you really are.

Second, humility is the choice to think less of yourself and more of others. C.S. Lewis put it this way: "True humility is not thinking less of yourself; it is thinking of yourself less." The more you focus on yourself and your own shabbiness, the less real you will feel. The more you focus on others and their needs, the more real you will feel.

Final thought

When you know deep down that you're loved and valued by God, yourself, and others, your shabbiness doesn't matter. Your exposed brokenness can become strength for others.

Detour Reflections

❖ What is your story of brokenness?

❖ What part of the story of *The Velveteen Rabbit* can you identify with?

Chapter 30: Impact

Impact is defined as "the effect or impression of one thing on another."[78] What effect have you had on others? What effect have others had on you? The possibilities for making a positive impact are endless.

Throughout my detour and season of re-entry, numerous people had a positive impact on my life. I also believe that I have had a positive effect on others. Choosing to make a positive impact was a tangible way to give something back for all I had received.

The legendary Jackie Robinson said, "A life is not important except in the impact it has on other lives." Below are just a few of the ways I found to have a positive impact on others.

Powerful ways to impact others

Adjust your perspective when entering a room from "Here I am!" to "There you are!"

Believe in the value and potential of people.

Call people by name and remember to smile.

Don't give up because life is hard—it will encourage others to do the same.

Envision yourself making an impact before you actually make it— doors will open as a result.

Forgive yourself and others.

Give unconditional love to others.

Help others carry loads too heavy for their shoulders.

Initiate conversations with open-ended questions (those that can't be answered with a yes or no).

Jump at the chance to thank others for what they've done.

Keep short accounts of the wrongs done to you.

Learn something new every day, and pass it on whenever possible.

Make a small difference every day—it will add up to a big difference over a lifetime.

Never use your words to put others down or spread disrespect.

Offer lonely people the time to hear their stories.

Pick up the pieces of a broken life without offering a quick fix.

Quiet your own soul first thing in the morning before entering a noisy world.

Raise the bar of expectation —it will help other people reach higher.

Say no to expectations you have no control over fulfilling.

Tell the truth when it helps others in the long run, not just to make you feel better.

Understand others before you expect them to understand you.

Value people by looking past their faults and weaknesses to see their potential.

Walk beside others who are hurting.

X-rays are like a discerning friend—they reveal inner brokenness so healing can occur.

Yard work done for you when you can't do it has a huge impact.

Zest for life is fueled by serving others.

Football great Ray Lewis said, "Don't walk through life just playing football. Don't walk through life just being an athlete. Athletics will fade. Character and integrity and really making an impact on someone's life, that's the ultimate vision, that's the ultimate goal."[79]

Compassion and impact

During my journey of re-entry, getting back into the mainstream of life, I often encountered people who were on their own detour. On one occasion, I told my story of the painful transition I had gone through and was now coming out of. After my talk, a cancer survivor came up and thanked me for what I had said. He also told me his story. His detour wasn't over, but he said he had received hope and encouragement from hearing my story. I was humbled to have been able to have an impact on his life.

As I walked away, I asked myself, "What was it about that visit that lit a fire inside me? Where did the joy I feel come from? Why do I feel a little bit more alive because our paths crossed?" The answer came when I started to understand how feeling my own pain in relation to someone else's pain actually can increase joy. Community and solidarity are at the heart of the movement from sorrow to joy. When you begin to feel your pain in relation to other people's pain, you can face it together. This is where the word compassion comes from—it means "to suffer with." When you share your experience of pain with somebody else, you can be compassionate.

This is how the healing begins—by experiencing the powerlessness of "not knowing what to do" together. As we feel the pain of our own losses, our hearts open to a wider world of suffering and loss; the pain in our life connects us with the moaning and groaning of a suffering humanity.[80]

As you fan the flame of compassion, you increase your capacity to impact others who are suffering. It is in that connection that you will find greater healing and wholeness.

How to know you are making a difference

During my detour, I asked myself this question: "Am I really making a difference in people's lives and impacting others for good?" I wasn't sure. When I was trying to re-engage with regular life, I asked the question again. Both times, my view of what was really going on was clouded by the feeling of being sidelined. Thankfully, I caught glimpses of the impact I was having on people and was encouraged greatly.

One story that helped to change my perspective was called "The Useless Tree." It goes like this: A carpenter and his apprentice were walking through a large forest. When they came across a tall, old tree, the carpenter asked his apprentice: "Do you know why this tree is so tall, so huge, so gnarled, so old, and so beautiful?" The apprentice answered, "No. Why?" The carpenter said,

"Because it is useless. If it had been useful, it would have been cut down long ago and made into tables and chairs. Because it is useless, it could grow so tall and so beautiful that you can sit in its shade and relax."[81]

Strong oak trees and beautiful diamonds are not created quickly or without enduring stress and harsh conditions. For long periods of time, the oak tree grows quietly in the forest and appears unproductive. But eventually it will provide shade for the weary traveler.

When I first stumbled onto this powerful image during my detour, I gained courage to be shade for weary travelers along the road even when I felt that I was doing very little. Later on, while I was working my way back into the mainstream of life, the image reminded me again of the impact I was continuing to have. To see myself as an old oak tree gave me courage and reminded me to appreciate where I'd come from and where I was.

Four lessons from the useless tree

1. Things are seldom as they appear.

Just when you think no one is watching or no one cares, out of nowhere a little voice says, "More is happening than you are even aware of." When I felt that the light of my life was contained within a walled room, I didn't see that I was having any impact. Then I would hear from a random source the difference I was making in someone's life.

2. If you focus only on "getting things done," you're only half right.

For much of my life, I had an unhealthy focus on production and "doing," which led to weakness, not greater strength. But going through times of waiting and struggle developed an inner strength of "being." Character does not develop within us if we are focused only on external production.

3. Without a certain amount of stress, growth is impossible.

A certain amount of stress is necessary in order for us to grow strong and stable. The oak tree that stands strong in the forest has withstood storms, wind, drought, and disease to grow stronger still. In life, the right amount of stress causes muscles to grow strong, diamonds to grow hard, character to develop, and beauty to be formed in our lives.

4. There is opportunity in calamity, not calamity in opportunity.

When you think of a tree that is left to age over time, it can look like a missed opportunity, but the reverse is actually true. Being left to endure the seasons and storms is the calamity that births opportunity. This truth is summarized powerfully in a prayer offered by the late Peter Marshall: "Our Father, when we long for life without trials and work, without difficulties, remind us that oaks grow strong in contrary winds and diamonds are made under pressure. With stout hearts may we see in every calamity an opportunity and not give way to the pessimist that sees in every opportunity a calamity."[82]

Final thoughts

As I look at all the ways others have impacted my life, I am filled with gratitude. I am also filled with gratitude as I think of the opportunities I've had to impact others. It isn't all about being productive and getting things done. It's also about showing up just as you are, with grace and peace, offering shade to weary travelers. When I take time to listen, connect, and be with those who suffer, life happens. It makes feeling useless worth it.

Detour Reflections

❖ How has your life been changed by the impact of others?

❖ What can you do today to have an impact on someone else?

Epilog: My New Road

Thanks for reading *Detour*. I hope you have found it informative, inspiring, and helpful as a roadmap for what you have been through, are going through, or will go through in the future.

In this final section, I tie up some of the loose ends left dangling in my story. I also provide some guidance so you can build on what you've learned and not lose the growth opportunity that awaits you as you travel detours of your own. I answer some basic questions you might have, such as: "What exactly is your new normal? What are you doing for work now? Where do I go from here? How can I stay in touch with you?"

What is my new normal life?

People who saw me during the detour ask me how I'm doing now. As tricky as it is to answer that, my answer is usually a description of my new normal. However, in order for me to talk about my new normal, it will be helpful for me to describe my old normal so you will have something to compare it to.

My normal before the accident was this: "I was an active fifty-year-old who was physically fit, bodily flexible, globally mobile, and growing as an international leadership coach and faster marathon runner." After the detour, I describe my new normal like this: "I'm a somewhat active fifty-six-year-old who is physically fit and bodily inflexible, a regionally based leadership coach and writer, and a person who cycles and walks for exercise."

Physically, I'm healthy, but I do live with mobility and stiffness issues. My right leg is two-and-a-half inches shorter than my left, requiring all my shoes (my runners, cycling shoes, golf shoes, sandals, water shoes, dress shoes, and casual shoes) to have an external lift mounted to the bottom of the sole to even things out.

My right quad and knee, which used to work perfectly before, work awkwardly now and are numb, tight, stiff, tingly, and puffed up. The bend in my right knee goes easily to 115 degrees, and the knee can be forced to bend up to 122 degrees. A normal knee can bend up to 150 degrees.

New normal bike riding starts out with my brain telling my knee to loosen up. In five to ten minutes, the knee obeys, and it cooperates for the rest of the ride. When I get out of the car, I appreciate a wide open door so I can get my knee out without lifting my leg three feet in the air.

If I walk too far, I wear myself out with sore knees and a shoulder that starts to ache when left in the hanging position too long. I can cycle for extended periods of time with little difficulty. If I sit too long, I stiffen up, which motivates me to stay active and get my daily bike ride in (indoors or out).

Mentally, I feel strong and resilient. I accept the role suffering plays in my life and the inevitability of its presence. The mental toughness I've developed helps me experiment with new ventures, face disappointment, and deal with setbacks and failure.

Vicky's Detour

My wife Vicky was my closest companion on my detour, but she was also on a detour of her own. During the accident, unlike me, she saw the car run the stop sign, heard my moans while I was under the engine block, and felt relief when she saw the Royal Columbian Hospital (RCH) crest on the paramedic's jacket.

What was her recovery like? She was flown with me by air ambulance to RCH, and she was also operated on that Easter Sunday morning. Her injuries included a broken femur and a broken forearm plus damage to her knee. The broken bones healed, but her knee continues to cause pain and discomfort, making it a challenge for her to walk and exercise.

Vicky left the hospital ten days after arriving and went to live with her parents until I arrived home on day 56. Her parents' home was equipped with a hospital bed, and she had regular visits from home care and the physiotherapist. Much of her time during those eight weeks was spent getting mobile again and visiting me.

Vicky went back to work ten months after the accident, to a modified role as a customer care representative. She reduced her hours from forty to thirty per week, a schedule which she continues today. Her companionship and support during those ten months before she went back to work made a huge difference as I continued with my recovery.

What work do I do now?

When people ask me what I do for work, I can't offer a clear-cut answer. The reason for that is that there is a wide range of services I perform and a great variety of ways I engage with people to help them—in the church, in non-profit organizations, and in the business arena.

In the months leading up to the accident, I had started to work with a US-based coaching company that provided leadership coaching and training to large corporate clients in the United States. I had my visa to work in the US and was on the bench as the next coach in line to step into the next project that came along. Then the accident happened.

In the weeks that followed the accident, I remained optimistic, believing that I would re-engage and bounce back in just a few months. Reality was very different. Instead of bouncing back, I faced the harsh reality of a recovery journey that lasted for years, not just months. The work in the US I had planned to get back to dried up, and I was left to consider other options.

After plenty of time to reflect on what I would do for meaningful work, I decided to sharpen my coaching skills for working with leaders and organizations both in the church and in the business arena. I became certified as an executive coach and went to work to expand my reach to those within driving distance of my home.

What do I do? I coach leaders one-on-one, support non-profits, facilitate strategic planning, host and facilitate collaborative conversations, coach teams, resource and train transitional pastors, publish books, speak, lead workshops, and lead a team of leaders within Outreach Canada. I'm an author who self-published *Between Pastors: Seizing the Opportunity*, with the help of Alan Simpson, after completing the book during my recovery. *Detour* is my second self-published book—and I am confident there will be more to come.

Another new pursuit I jumped into at the tail end of my recovery was to join Toastmasters International. This came about thanks to the prodding of my Uncle Ross. He is a seasoned Toastmaster, and he challenged me to use Toastmasters to hone my speaking skills and to better equip myself to tell my story to the world. I'm two years in and am seeing meaningful fruit from the investment I have made.

Where to from here?

The future is bright and filled with possibilities. Remarkable people have helped me each step of the way, and I want to do the same for others. I get up every morning and live out my purpose with as much intentionality and focus as I can. When I fall, I pick up a few things while I'm down there, then get up to try again.

Motorcycle riding has been replaced by tandem cycling. Running has been replaced by walking and mountain biking. Life includes struggle, pleasure, loss, adventure, sorrow, laughter, reflection, action, and learning to embrace the full gamut of human experience.

I invite you to put into practice what you've learned in this book. I've created the *Detour Journal* to help you track your growth, record your insights, process your emotions, and transform your life. I invite you to visit my website www.camtaylor.net, where you can join my email list, order your copy of the *Detour Journal*, and receive ongoing support and inspiration for your journey.

My purpose is to help people find their why and their way. I hope this book has helped you to do both. I look forward to hearing from you. I would especially like to hear how this book has helped you on your journey. And, if you have received help, please tell your friends so they, too, can be encouraged and supported on their journey.

May your future be bright —not because you have wishful thinking but because you have true hope and a pathway to see that hope realized.

Appendix: Statistics

Hospital stays

April 23-May 13, 2011: Royal Columbian Hospital, 21 days
May 13-20, 2011: Abbotsford Hospital, 7 days
May 20-June 2, 2011: Worthington Pavilion, 14 days
June 2-18, 2011: Bevan Lodge, 16 days
September 5-17, 2011: Royal Columbian Hospital, 13 days
November 9-19, 2011: Royal Columbian Hospital, 11 days
February 2-6, 2012: Royal Columbian Hospital, 5 days
May 1-5, 2012: Royal Columbian Hospital, 5 days
October 22-25, 2012: Royal Columbian Hospital, 4 days
January 20-26, 2014: Royal Columbian Hospital, 7 days

Surgery dates and details

April 24, 2011: dealt with my broken femur, tibia, and upper arm
May 1, 2011: inserted a suction pump to help remove infection
May 3, 2011: removed the suction pump and closed up the leg wound
September 8, 2011: opened up my leg and removed infected bone chips and tissue
November 9, 2011: opened up my leg and removed six inches of infected femur; attached an external fixator to hold the remaining femur in place; placed a cement spacer to fill the gap where the removed femur had been; restarted antibiotics
February 2, 2012: opened up the quad muscle; removed the external fixator; inserted a rod; continued with antibiotics
May 1, 2012: attached the bone transporter to my right femur
October 22, 2012: removed the bone transporter; started the continuous passive motion machine
January 20, 2014: knee release and quadricepsplasty

July 7, 2015: removed the hardware in my right upper arm (day surgery)

Other statistics

- Total number of staples used in surgeries – 484
- Total number of sutures used in surgeries – 46
- Days I couldn't drive: 717 days
- Hours in the recliner: more than 5000 hours
- Weeks on antibiotics: 6 weeks X 4 rounds = 24 weeks

Acknowledgments

I begin by thanking God for being my constant traveling companion each step of the way. I learned so much about how God works and who He really is. I'm grateful to have been given a few more years to live out my purpose here on earth. My faith and character have definitely grown, thanks to God's watchful attentiveness during this process.

I thank my family, who were there from day one, especially Vicky, whose love and support were tireless. She cried with me, laughed with me, sat with me, taxied me, cared for me, and helped carry the load with me. I thank my kids, Caleb and Elena, who were there to greet me when I opened my eyes in the ICU and cheered me on each step of the way.

I thank my parents, Keith and Joan Taylor, for teaching me the lessons I would put into practice during my detour. They also helped carry me along during the detour with their prayers, visits, and encouragement. I thank my sisters, Beth and Marilou, and Vicky's siblings, Nancy and John, for their steady love and constant contact throughout the journey.

I thank Vicky's parents, Eugene and Helen Parkins, who put their lives on hold to look after us with rides, meals, housing, visits, and abundant support. I thank Garry and Shirlene Henning, who went from basement tenants to basement caring family. I also thank our lifelong friends, Rob and Debbie Deyo, who supported Vicky and me with love, companionship, and timely nursing care.

I thank the paramedics, the volunteer firefighters, the helicopter pilot, the police officers, the neighbor with the floor jack, the owner of the lap I laid my head on while lying on the road, and the community who came to our rescue. I never had the chance to properly thank you.

A huge debt of gratitude goes to everyone at Royal Columbian Hospital (RCH), who did what they do best—help people in trauma. Thanks to the orthopedic surgeons, GPs, hospitalists, anesthesiologists, infectious disease specialists, nurses, care aids, physiotherapists, occupational therapists, and many other staff members who made the healing process possible. Thanks go to Dr. Bertrand Perry, who, along with his team, put Vicky and me back together when we first arrived. I am very grateful for the skillful hands of surgeon Dr. Darius Viskontas, who took over my case when it became complicated and I required reconstructive surgery.

Thanks to the countless professionals and support workers who were there to help when we came home—the home care workers, the house cleaners, the occupational therapists, the physiotherapists, the case workers, the lawyers, the insurance specialists, the taxi drivers, my psychotherapist, and our family doctor.

Thanks to friends and family who fed me, pushed me in my wheelchair, let me use their electric scooter, drove me to appointments, mowed my lawn, brought me barbecue chips, cried with me, sat in silence, made me laugh, and walked beside me. I thank my neighbors, who created a cone of support whenever I went out of the house for some fresh air.

I thank my Outreach Canada family, who prayed, visited, covered for me, and walked beside me throughout the journey. I thank my New Heights Church family for their prayers, their support, and a platform where I shared my struggle.

I thank those who mentored and encouraged me through books, podcasts, TED Talks, movies, DVDs, YouTube videos, and personal visits. I thank the thousands I never met from all over the world who heard our story and prayed for us. I'm humbled just thinking about it.

Getting this book to print was a team effort. I thank my Mom for her many edits, corrections, and faithful proofreading efforts. I thank my editor, James R. Coggins, whose well-trained eye helped shape the manuscript into what it became. I thank Bitty Berlinghoff for her creativity and skill in designing the cover. Thanks also to my many blog readers, who gave me input as I told my story while it was being lived.

And to all of you who read this book, thank you for sharing the journey with me. My hope and prayer is that whether your detour is behind you, you are on one now, or you anticipate one in the future, you will find hope and help for the journey.

Endnotes

[1] Ecclesiastes 3:1-4, NIV.

[2] Nelson Mandela, *Long Walk to Freedom* (New York: Little, Brown and Company, 2008), Location 8927-8928, Kindle edition.

[3] *Collins English Dictionary: Complete and Unabridged*, s.v. "complain," retrieved July 17, 2016, http://www.thefreedictionary.com/ complain

[4] Viktor E. Frankl, *Man's Search for Meaning* (Boston: Beacon Press, 1959), 97-99.

[5] Genesis 2:18, NIV.

[6] *Wikipedia*, s.v. "Carpe diem," last modified July 29, 2016, https://en.wikipedia.org/wiki/Carpe_diem

[7] I first heard about this idea in Stephen Covey's book, *Seven Habits of Highly Effective People* (New York: Simon and Schuster, 1989).

[8] Daniel Pink, "The Power of Habits—and the Power to Change Them," accessed August 18, 2016, http://www.danpink.com/2012/03/the-power-of-habits-and-the-power-to-change-them/

[9] *American Heritage Dictionary of the English Language*, 5th ed. (Houghton Mifflin Harcourt, 2016), s.v. "endurance," retrieved January 19, 2017, http://www.thefreedictionary.com/endurance.

[10] Danutz, "John Stephen Akhwari—Inspirational Story," accessed August 18, 2016, http://www.athslife.com/2014/05/john-stephen-akhwari/

[11] *Wikipedia*, s.v. "Anesthesia," last modified August 11, 2016, https://en.wikipedia.org/wiki/Anesthesia

[12] Dennis N.T. Perkins, *Leading at the Edge: Leadership Lessons from the Extraordinary Saga of Shackleton's Antarctic Expedition*, 2nd ed. (New York: American Management Association, 2012), 19, Kindle edition.

[13] Perkins, *Leading at the Edge*, 24.

[14] Coco Brooks, "Clark Family," accessed August 18, 2016, https://www.cocobrooks.com/box-stories/clark-family

[15] International Kiko Goat Association, "Goat Jokes," accessed August 18, 2016, http://www.theikga.org/goat_jokes.html

[16] Harvey Schachter, "Managing Books: Nine key traits to make the shift from failure to success," accessed August 18, 2016, http://www.theglobeandmail.com/report-on-business/careers/management/nine-key-traits-to-make-the-shift-from-failure-to-success/article4598952/

[17] Schachter, "Managing Books."

[18] *Dictionary.com: Unabridged,* s.v. "resilience," accessed January 18, 2016, http://www.dictionary.com/browse/adversity.

[19] Robert Luckadoo, *Grit in your Craw* (Jackson, MS: Southern Flair Communications, 2016), Location 881, Kindle edition.

[20] *Dictionary.com: Unabridged,* s.v. "adversity," accessed September 8, 2016, http://www.dictionary.com/browse/adversity

[21] Romans 8:28, NLT.

[22] James 1:2-4, MSG.

[23] Aimee Mullins, "The Opportunity of Adversity," TED video, 21:58, filmed in October 2009, http://www.ted.com/talks/aimee_mullins_the_opportunity_of_adversity

[24] J.D. Meier, "Dr. Normal Rosenthal on 7 Tricks for Dealing with Adversity," accessed September 11, 2016, http://sourcesofinsight.com/dr-normal-rosenthal-on-7-tricks-for-dealing-with-adversity/

[25] *Collins English Dictionary – Complete and Unabridged, 10th ed.,* s.v. "emotion," accessed September 11, 2016, http://www.dictionary.com/browse/emotion

[26] Steven J. Stein and Howard E. Book, *The EQ Edge: Emotional Intelligence and Your Success* (San Francisco: Jossey-Bass, 2011), 58.

[27] *Wikipedia,* s.v. "Serenity Prayer," last modified July 11, 2016, https://en.wikipedia.org/wiki/Serenity_Prayer

[28] Robert Browning Hamilton, "Quotes," Goodreads (blog), accessed September 11, 2016, http://www.goodreads.com/quotes/289683-i-walked-a-mile-with-pleasure-she-chatted-all-the

[29] Philip Yancey, *Where Is God When It Hurts?* (Grand Rapids, MI: Zondervan, 2002), 37.

[30] G.K. Chesterton, "Orthodoxy Quotes," Goodreads (blog), accessed September 11, 2016, https://www.goodreads.com/work/quotes/1807543-orthodoxy

[31] *Dictionary.com: Unabridged,* c.v. "grief," accessed September 11, 2016, http://www.dictionary.com/browse/grief

[32] Psalm 66:12, NIV.

[33] Debra Stang, "The 4 Tasks of Grief," accessed September 11, 2016, http://www.allianceofhope.org/blog_/2012/07/the-4-tasks-of-grief.html

[34] University of South Florida, "Is Crying a Good Thing? Maybe. Sometimes," last modified December 10, 2008, http://news.usf.edu/article/templates/?a=1038

35 Psalm 56:8, MSG.

36 Lou LaGrand, "Why Crying is Coping and Why You Should Cry If You Can," Ezinearticles, accessed July 27, 2016, http://ezinearticles.com/?Why-Crying-is-Coping-and-Why-You-Should-Cry-If-You-Can&id=601878

37 Genesis 50:19-20, NLT.

38 *The American Heritage Dictionary of the English Language, 5th ed., s.v.* "perseverance," accessed September 11, 2016, http://www.thefreedictionary.com/perseverance

39 Henry Cloud, "Dr Cloud Daily," email message to Cam Taylor, September 2, 2016.

40 Brad Gast, "Never Stop Believing," The Daily Quotes (blog), accessed September 11, 2016, http://thedailyquotes.com/tag/brad-gast/

41 Haruki Murakami, "Quotes," Goodreads (blog), accessed September 11, 2016, https://www.goodreads.com/author/quotes/3354. Haruki_Murakami

42 Aimee Mullins, "The Opportunity of Adversity," TED Partner Series, accessed January 26, 2017, http://empowermentthroughopportunity.com/Aimee%20Mullins%20-%20The%20Opportunity%20of%20Adversity.pdf

43 Proverbs 14:30, NIV.

44 Dr. Seuss, "Oh, The Places You'll Go!" Nooch Net, accessed September 26, 2016, http://denuccio.net/ohplaces.html

45 *Wikipedia*, s.v. "Dayenu," last modified February 25, 2016, https://en.wikipedia.org/wiki/Dayenu

46 Jeff Manion, *The Land Between: Finding God in Difficult Transitions* (Grand Rapids, MI: Zondervan, 2010), 9.

47 *Wikipedia*, s.v. "Koinonia," last modified April 14, 2016, https://en.wikipedia.org/wiki/Koinonia

48 Kate Torgovnick May, "I am, because of you: Further reading on Ubuntu," TED blog, accessed September 11, 2016, http://blog.ted.com/further-reading-on-ubuntu/

49 *Collins English Dictionary – Complete and Unabridged, 12th ed. 2014, s.v.* "discipline," accessed July 27, 2016, http://www.thefreedictionary.com/discipline

50 *The American Heritage Dictionary of the English Language, 5th ed., s.v.* "remember," accessed September 11, 2016, http://www.thefreedictionary.com/remember

51 Margaret Farley Steele, "Making Sense of Senseless Violence," *HealthDay*, July 27, 2016, https://consumer.healthday.com/kids-health-

information-23/parenting-health-news-525/making-sense-of-senseless-violence-712961.html

[52] Henri Nouwen, "Care, The Source of All Cure," Windows Toward the World (blog), January 8, 2012, https://helenl.wordpress.com/2012/01/08/care-the-source-of-all-cure-henri-nouwen/

[53] *The American Heritage® Stedman's Medical Dictionary*, s.v. "cure," accessed March 13, 2017, http://www.dictionary.com/browse/cure

[54] Jim Collins and Morten T. Hansen, *Great by Choice: Uncertainty, Chaos, and Luck – Why Some Thrive Despite Them All* (New York: Harper Business, 2011), 13-15.

[55] Nelson Mandela, *Long Walk to Freedom*, Location 3049, Kindle edition.

[56] James M. Kouzes and Barry Z. Posner, *The Leadership Challenge, 4th ed.* (San Francisco: Jossey-Bass, 2007), 203.

[57] "Be a Hummingbird, Not a Vulture," Better Life Coaching (blog), July 1, 2011, https://betterlifecoachingblog.com/2011/07/01/be-a-hummingbird-not-a-vulture/

[58] *English Oxford Living Dictionaries*, s.v. "work," accessed April 17, 2017, https://en.oxforddictionaries.com/definition/us/work

[59] Terry Bacon and Karen Spear, *Adaptive Coaching: The Art and Practice of a Client-Centered Approach to Performance Improvement* (Boston: Nicholas Brealey America, 2003), 307-324.

[60] William Arthur Ward, "To Risk," Growing Up (blog), March 20, 2006, http://mikechandler.blogspot.ca/2006/03/i-love-this-poem-to-risk.html

[61] Bacon and Spear, *Adaptive Coaching*, 312-315.

[62] Matt Long, *The Long Run: One Man's Attempt to Regain His Athletic Career – And His Life – by Running the New York City Marathon* (Rodale Books, 2010). To find out more, go to http://www.goodreads.com/book/show/8343757-the-long-run

[63] 2 Minute Insight, Summary: *Mindset: The New Psychology of Success* – the Optimist's Summary of Carol Dweck's Best Selling Book (2 Minute Insight, 2014), Location 79, Kindle edition.

[64] 1 Samuel 17.

[65] 2 Minute Insight, *Mindset*, Location 248, Kindle edition.

[66] Seth Godin, *The Icarus Deception: How High Will You Fly?* (London: Porfolio, 2012), 47.

[67] Henry Cloud's advice quoted in this chapter comes from his Daily Dr Cloud: www.drcloud.com

[68] Steven Pressfield, *The War of Art: Break Through the Blocks and Win Your Inner Creative Battles* (New York: Black Irish Entertainment, 2002), Location 162, Kindle edition.

⁶⁹ Pressfield, *The War of Art*, Location 178.

⁷⁰ Proverbs 18:21, MSG.

⁷¹ Proverbs 25:11, MSG.

⁷² Quizlet, s.v. "momentum," accessed March 14, 2017, https://quizlet.com/163166251/forces-flash-cards/

⁷³ Lorii Myers, "Quotes About Momentum," Goodreads (blog), accessed July 28, 2016, http://www.goodreads.com/quotes/tag/momentum

⁷⁴ *Dictionary.com: Unabridged*, s.v. "opportunity," accessed September 3, 2015, http://www.dictionary.com/browse/opportunity

⁷⁵ Seth Godin, "Burning Questions With Seth Godin: Faith, Lizards, and Your Art," Danielle Laporte (blog), accessed September 13, 2016, http://www.daniellelaporte.com/burning-questions-with-seth-godin-faith-lizards-and-your-art/

⁷⁶ Covey, *Seven Habits*, 69.

⁷⁷ Margery Williams, "The Velveteen Rabbit," accessed March 29, 2004, http://archive.org/stream/thevelveteenrabb11757gut/11757.txt

⁷⁸ *The Free Dictionary*, s.v. "impact," accessed March 15, 2017, http://www.thefreedictionary.com/impact

⁷⁹ Ray Lewis, "Ray Lewis Quotes," Brainy Quote, accessed September 13, 2016, http://www.brainyquote.com/quotes/quotes/r/raylewis480999.html

⁸⁰ Henri Nouwen, *Spiritual Formation: Following the Movements of the Spirit* (Toronto: HarperCollins Publishing, 2010), Location 916-924, Kindle edition.

⁸¹ Nouwen, *Spiritual Formation*, Location 556.

⁸² George O. Wood, *A Psalm in Your Heart* (Springfield, MI: Gospel Publishing House, 2008), Location 4920, Kindle edition.